A Manual for Writers

Chicago Guides
to *Writing*, Editing*
and Publishing

On Writing, Editing, and Publishing
Jacques Barzun

Getting into Print
Walter W. Powell

Writing for Social Scientists
Howard S. Becker

Chicago Guide for Preparing
Electronic Manuscripts
Prepared by the Staff of the
University of Chicago Press

Tales of the Field
John Van Maanen

A Handbook of
Biological Illustration
Frances W. Zweifel

The Craft of Translation
John Biguenet and
Rainer Schulte, editors

Style
Joseph M. Williams

Mapping It Out
Mark Monmonier

Indexing Books
Nancy C. Mulvany

Writing Ethnographic Fieldnotes
Robert M. Emerson, Rachel I.
Fretz, and Linda L. Shaw

Glossary of Typesetting Terms
Richard Eckersley, Richard
Angstadt, Charles M. Ellerston,
Richard Hendel, Naomi B.
Pascal, and Anita Walker Scott

The Craft of Research
Wayne C. Booth, Gregory G.
Colomb, and Joseph M. Williams

A Poet's Guide to Poetry
Mary Kinzie

A Manual for Writers of Term Papers, Theses, and Dissertations

Kate L. Turabian

Sixth Edition
Revised by
John Grossman and Alice Bennett

The University of Chicago Press
Chicago and London

Portions of this book have been adapted from *The Chicago Manual of Style*, 14th edition, © 1969, 1982, 1993 by The University of Chicago, and from *A Manual for Writers of Term Papers, Theses, and Dissertations* by Kate L. Turabian, revised and expanded for the fifth edition by Bonnie Birtwistle Honigsblum.

The University of Chicago Press, Chicago 60637
The University of Chicago Press, Ltd., London

04 03   5 6 7 8 9 10

ISBN: 0-226-81626-5 (cloth)
       0-226-81627-3 (paper)

                Library of Congress Cataloging-in-Publication Data

Turabian, Kate L.
    A manual for writers of term papers, theses, and dissertations / Kate L. Turabian.—6th ed. / rev. by John Grossman and Alice Bennett.
        p.   cm.—(Chicago guides to writing, editing, and publishing)
    Includes bibliographical references and index.
    1. Dissertations, Academic.   2. Report writing.   I. Grossman, John, 1924–   II. Bennett, Alice, 1938–   III. Title.   IV. Series.
LB2369.T8   1996
808'.02—dc20   95-43267
                                                                    CIP

Contents

Preface   vii

1   Parts of the Paper   1

2   Abbreviations and Numbers   14

3   Spelling and Punctuation   39

4   Capitalization, Italics, and Quotation Marks   64

5   Quotations   73

6   Tables   87

7   Illustrations   104

8   Notes   116

9   Bibliographies   165

10   Parenthetical References and Reference Lists   175

11   Comparing the Two Documentation Systems   185

12   Public Documents   214

13   Preparing the Manuscript   239

14   Formats and Sample Layouts   251

         Selected Bibliography   283

         Index   287

Preface

Kate L. Turabian designed this manual as a guide to suitable style for presenting formal papers—term papers, theses, dissertations—in the humanities, social sciences, and natural sciences. Over the course of sixty years the book has become established as one of the basic reference works for undergraduate and graduate students in many disciplines. This sixth edition has been prompted by publication of the fourteenth edition of *The Chicago Manual of Style* and by new guidelines on dissertations from the Office of Academic Publications at the University of Chicago.

The University of Chicago Press receives many inquiries about Kate Turabian and the history of her manual. A reviewer for *Quill and Scroll* wrote that Turabian's name had become "part of the folklore of American higher education," and she has been called "the Emily Post of scholarship." So legendary has she become that some believe she is an invention. In fact, Kate Turabian worked for over thirty years at the University of Chicago, where she was dissertation secretary from 1930 to 1958. She died in 1987 at age ninety-four, a few months after publication of the fiftieth anniversary edition of her manual. Commenting on the more than eleven thousand theses and dissertations she inspected for the university, she told the *Chicago Tribune,* "I learned early that modern young people have ideas of their own on grammar and punctuation." It was to correct and guide these ideas that she wrote the instruction sheets that were given out to graduate students at the university. She later adapted materials from the Press's *Manual of Style* to expand the guidelines into a sixty-eight-page booklet, copyrighted by the University of Chicago in 1937 and distributed first by the campus bookstore, then by the Press. The University of Chicago Press published the book under its own imprint in a revised edition issued in 1955. Three years later Kate Turabian retired as dissertation secretary, but she remained involved in the next two revisions of her manual, published in 1967 and 1973. The fifth edition, substantially revised and enlarged by

Bonnie Honigsblum, was published in 1987. This sixth edition has been revised by John Grossman, now retired as managing editor of the University of Chicago Press, who also prepared the fourteenth edition of *The Chicago Manual of Style,* and by Alice Bennett, senior manuscript editor at the Press.

From the beginning Kate Turabian's book has had a close connection with the Press's older style manual. Since the tenth edition of the Press's manual was published in 1937, each new edition has been followed by a revision of "Turabian." This sixth edition brings Turabian's manual into conformity with the fourteenth edition of *The Chicago Manual of Style.* The new edition also reflects changes brought about by the increasing use of personal computers for preparing research papers. When Turabian's manual was last revised in 1987, many students were still using typewriters. Those who worked with computers found that word processing programs were not designed for the special formatting requirements of scholarly papers, such as placing footnotes at the bottom of the page. In less than a decade, the situation has changed dramatically. Not only do many more students have access to computers, but software now addresses the particular needs of scholars and students and offers a typographic sophistication that was not available before. With the help of style sheets, students can reduce the time spent on formatting and concentrate on presenting ideas. Dissertation offices can allow greater flexibility in decisions regarding margins, spacing, emphasis, headings, and general presentation. This new environment is reflected in the current edition, especially in chapter 13 on manuscript preparation and in chapter 14, showing sample pages from typical research papers.

Regular users of this manual will find that its basic structure remains much the same as in the fifth edition. Some chapters have been retitled or rearranged, but the same major topics are covered. Chapter 1 describes the parts of a long formal paper. Chapters 2–5 introduce students to the mechanics of writing, including the use of abbreviations, the treatment of numbers, some principles of spelling, punctuation, capitalization, and the use of italics, and the way to present quotations. Chapters 6 and 7 show how to prepare and refer to tables and illustrations. The section on documentation, chapters 8–12, describes two of the most commonly used systems of citation—the humanities style using notes and bibliographical references and the author-date style favored by scholars in the social and natural sciences—and gives many examples.

It is not within the scope of this manual to offer advice on how to select a topic, undertake research, and write up the results. That challenge is taken up by three master teachers, Wayne C. Booth, Gregory G. Colomb, and Joseph M. Williams, in their recent book *The Craft of Research* (Chicago, 1995), which is intended as a companion to Turabian's manual. Students may also need to consult a specialized style manual prescribed by their academic department or discipline. Although many scholarly authors and publishers follow one of the methods of documentation described here, there is not universal acceptance of every detail. Some disciplines follow the citation style of manuals published by learned societies or scholarly journals, listed in the bibliography at the end of this book.

The revisers of this edition thank all those who contributed information useful to the preparation of the fifth and sixth editions of Turabian's *Manual.* These include the many teachers, dissertation secretaries, and thesis advisers who have written to the Press with suggestions or have answered questionnaires, as well as members of the University of Chicago community who have advised on various items. The revisers have endeavored to continue Turabian's tradition of selecting the parts of *The Chicago Manual of Style* that are most useful to students.

1 Parts of the Paper

Introduction 1.1
Front Matter, or Preliminaries 1.7
  ⸱ Title Page 1.7
  Blank Page or Copyright Page 1.8
  Dedication 1.9
  Epigraph 1.10
  ⸱Table of Contents 1.11
  List of Illustrations 1.19
  List of Tables 1.24
  Preface 1.25
  Acknowledgments 1.26
  List of Abbreviations 1.27
  Glossary 1.28
  Editorial Method 1.31
  Abstract 1.32
Text 1.33
  Introduction 1.34
  Part 1.35
  Chapter 1.36
  Section and Subsection 1.37
Back Matter, or Reference Matter 1.39
  Appendix 1.39
  Endnotes 1.46
  Bibliography or Reference List 1.47

INTRODUCTION

1.1   The word *paper* is used throughout this manual for term papers, theses, and dissertations except when referring specifically to one of these. A term paper fulfills one of the requirements of a course or an undergraduate major. A thesis is a requirement of a graduate-level course or a master's degree. A dissertation is one of the requirements for a doctorate. Each kind of research paper must include references giving full publication data for works cited in the text, and each is to be submitted as finished copy rather than as a manuscript prepared for typesetting. Before beginning work on such a research paper, the writer should consult the department or degree-granting institution to determine any special requirements. To the extent that these do not conflict with the guidelines offered in this manual, or if no special requirements exist, the style presented here is recommended.

1.2   All the basic text in a dissertation must be double-spaced, and double-spacing is strongly urged for all academic papers. Indented block quotations (5.30–34), however, may be single-spaced. It is also conventional to single-space footnotes, itemized lists, and bibliographies or reference lists, leaving a blank line between notes, items, or entries. Runover lines in tables of contents, lists of tables and illustrations, and subheads may also be single-spaced.

1.3   A paper has three main parts: the front matter, or preliminaries; the text; and the back matter or reference matter. In a long paper, each of these parts may consist of several sections (see below), each beginning a new page.

1.4   There are two categories of pagination: the front matter, numbered with consecutive lowercase roman numerals, centered at the bottom of the page, and the rest of the work, numbered with arabic numerals centered at the bottom of pages that bear titles and centered at the top (or placed in the upper right corner) of all other pages of the text and back matter.

1.5   Although all pages are counted in the pagination, some of the preliminaries do not have page numbers typed on them (see 1.7–11).

1.6   Unless specified otherwise by the conventions of a department or discipline, the order given in the table of contents for this chapter should be observed, though not every paper will require all these parts. Should the paper later be published, the organization required by the publisher may differ from that recommended here.

FRONT MATTER, OR PRELIMINARIES

TITLE PAGE

1.7 Many universities and colleges have their own style of title page for theses and dissertations, and this should be followed exactly for content, capitalization, and position and spacing of the elements. For term papers, if a sample sheet is not provided, a title page might include the name of the university or college (usually centered near the top of the sheet), the full title of the paper, the course (including its department and number), the date, and the name of the writer. Although the title page counts as page i, the number is not shown on it. See sample 14.18 for one style that may be used for theses and dissertations.

BLANK PAGE OR COPYRIGHT PAGE

1.8 A blank sheet prevents the text of the following page from showing through the white space on the title page. The sheet may also be used as a copyright page, with the copyright notice, in the following form, placed near the bottom.

```
Copyright © 19– by Arthur Author
     All rights reserved
```

In either case the sheet is counted in the pagination, but the page number is not shown. A copyright notice may be included even if the copyright is not registered.

DEDICATION

1.9 Dedications are usually brief and need not include the word *dedicated. To* is sufficient:

```
To Gerald
```

It is not necessary to identify (or even give the whole name of) the person to whom the work is dedicated or to give such other information as life dates, though both are permissible. Extravagant dedications are a thing of the past, and humorous ones rarely stand the test of time. The dedication, typed in uppercase and lowercase, should be centered on the width of a line about three inches from the top of the page, with no final punctuation. If *to* introduces the dedication, it should begin with a capital. A dedication is not listed in the table of contents. No number appears on it, but the page is counted in the pagination of the preliminaries.

EPIGRAPH

1.10 An epigraph—a quotation placed at the beginning of a work or of one of its parts and adumbrating its theme—is not italicized, underlined, or put in quotation marks. When an epigraph heads a whole paper, its format is like that of a dedication (see 1.9). For epigraphs that begin chapters or sections of a paper, see 5.9. The source is given on the line following the quotation and should consist only of the author's name (just the last name of a well-known author) and, usually, the title of the work. The title should be italicized or underlined or enclosed in quotation marks in accordance with the guidelines in chapter 4. Epigraphs are usually self-explanatory: any explanation should be included in the preface or other introductory matter. An epigraph is not listed in the table of contents. No number appears on it, but the page is counted in the pagination of the preliminaries.

TABLE OF CONTENTS

1.11 The table of contents, usually headed simply CONTENTS (in full capitals), lists all the parts of the paper except the title page, blank page or copyright page, dedication, and epigraph, which all precede it. No page numbers appear on any of these four, but all are counted in the pagination of the front matter. If the chapters are grouped in parts, the generic headings (e.g., PART I) and titles (e.g., EARLY FINDINGS) of the parts also appear in the contents, though the pages carry no numbers in the text (see 1.18). Subheads within the chapters are frequently included in one of various ways (see 14.19–20), or they may be omitted from the table of contents.

1.12 In preparing a table of contents for a paper containing one level or more of subheads (see 1.37), there is great latitude in both the amount of information included and the method of presenting it. At one extreme the contents may provide what is essentially an outline by including all the levels. At the other extreme the contents may omit the subheads—even though the paper carries subheads of one level or more than one—showing only the generic headings and titles of chapters. For many papers, both those with only one level and those with more than one level of subhead, the table of contents includes the first-level (principal) subheads, with or without the page numbers (sample 14.19). Note that when more than one level of subhead is included in the contents, they must appear in order of rank; that is, it is not permissible to begin with any but the first-level subhead or to skip from the first to the third or fourth level (sample 14.20).

1.13   First to be listed in the table of contents (see 14.19) are those elements of the front matter that have page numbers shown (1.19–32). These may include a list of illustrations, list of tables, preface, acknowledgments, list of abbreviations, glossary, editorial method, and abstract, usually in that order. Following the preliminaries, the various elements of the text are listed. Chapters are listed under that generic heading, with chapter numbers aligned at the left and chapter titles aligned on the first letter. If the chapters are divided into groups, or *parts,* the part title and number are centered above the constituent chapters (14.19). The back matter, or reference matter (appendix, endnotes, and bibliography or reference list; see 1.39–47), is listed last (14.20) and, like the front matter, starts flush left. A line space should be left between items in the table of contents; that is, the items are double-spaced. If an item runs to more than one line, however, the runover lines are single-spaced.

1.14   Subheads, when included, are indented a consistent distance (three spaces, for example) beyond the beginning of the chapter title. If more than one level of subhead is included, each level is indented an additional three spaces. Runovers are indented yet another three spaces, and the spaced periods (leaders) running to the page number (see 1.18) begin at the end of the last runover line. Multiple levels of subheads and a runover subhead are illustrated in example 14.20. If the subheads are short, those of the same level may be run in (run together), with each level, as a block, indented three spaces beyond the preceding one. Run-in subheads may be separated by semicolons, dashes, or periods.

1.15   Capitalization and wording of the titles of all parts, chapters, and sections should appear exactly as in the body of the paper.

1.16   Capitalization of titles in both the table of contents and the body of the paper should be as follows. For the titles of all major divisions (acknowledgments, preface, contents, list of illustrations, list of tables, list of abbreviations, glossary, editorial method, abstract, introduction, parts, chapters, appendix, notes, and bibliography or reference list), capitalize all letters (e.g., PREFACE). For subheads, use *headline style* (see 4.6–8), capitalizing the initial letter of the first and last words and of all other words except articles, prepositions, and coordinate conjunctions (sample 14.19), or use *sentence style* (see 4.9), capitalizing only the initial letter of the subhead and of any proper nouns or proper adjectives (sample 14.20).

1.17   Numbers designating parts and chapters should be given as they appear in the text. Part numbers may be uppercase roman numerals (PART I, PART II, etc.) or spelled-out numbers (PART ONE, PART TWO, etc.). The generic heading may precede the part title on the same line, followed by a period (sample 14.19), or it may be centered above the title and thus need no following punctuation (sample 14.20). Chapter numbers may be arabic or uppercase roman numerals or spelled-out numbers. The word *chapter* may precede each chapter number, or it may be given only once as a heading above the column listing all the chapter numbers (samples 14.19–20).

1.18   Page numbers in a table of contents are usually aligned on the right following a line of spaced periods (leaders) separating the title from the page number on which the part of the paper begins (sample 14.20). Note that only the *beginning* page number of each chapter or other section is given. Page numbers for parts need be given only if the part-title page contains some introductory text, but if the page number is given for one part, it must be given for all. Page numbers for subheads may be omitted (sample 14.19). When they are included with run-in subheads, page numbers are best placed in parentheses immediately following each subhead.

LIST OF ILLUSTRATIONS

1.19   In a list of illustrations, headed simply ILLUSTRATIONS, the figure numbers are given in arabic numerals followed by a period;

the captions follow the period; and the page numbers (in arabic) are usually separated from the caption by leaders. Double-space between captions, single-space within.

1.20 The figure numbers in the list are aligned on their periods under the word *figure,* and page numbers are listed flush right under the word *page,* as in sample 14.21.

1.21 Figures must not be numbered 1a, 1b, and so forth. A figure may, however, have lettered parts to which its legend, or descriptive statement, refers.

> Fig. 1. *Digitalis: a,* cross section of stem; *b,*
> enlargement of a seed.

Do not include the lettered parts in the list of illustrations.

1.22 The captions in the list of illustrations should agree with those given beneath the illustrations, unless the latter are long (more properly, then, called *legends*), in which case it is best to shorten them in the list. For a thesis or dissertation, however, consult the dissertation office. Even if a descriptive or explanatory statement follows the caption under an illustration, do not include it in the list of illustrations (sample 14.21).

1.23 In this list captions are capitalized headline style (see 4.6–8), as in sample 14.21. Foreign language captions, however, should follow the conventions for the language.

LIST OF TABLES

1.24 In a list of tables, the table numbers are arabic numerals followed by periods and are aligned on the periods in a left-hand column headed *table;* the page numbers are listed flush right under the heading *page.* The table titles begin two spaces after the period following the table number and should agree exactly with the titles above the tables themselves. The titles are capitalized either sentence or headline style (see 4.6–9), and runover lines are indented three spaces. Double-space between items, single-space within (sample 14.22).

PREFACE

1.25 In the preface, the writer explains the motivation for the study, the background of the project, the scope of the research, and the purpose of the paper. The preface may also include acknowledgments. If a writer has nothing significant to add to what is covered in the body of the paper and wishes only to acknowledge the various sorts of assistance and permissions received, these remarks should be titled ACKNOWLEDGMENTS rather than PREFACE. A preface appears in the same format as an acknowledgments section (see 1.26).

ACKNOWLEDGMENTS

1.26 In the acknowledgments, the writer thanks mentors and colleagues, lists the individuals or institutions that supported the research, and gives credit to works cited in the text for which permission to reproduce has been granted (see 5.1). Although one might wish to acknowledge special assistance such as consultation on technical matters or aid in securing special equipment and source materials, one may properly omit formal thanks for the routine help given by an adviser or a thesis committee. The generic heading ACKNOWLEDGMENTS, which appears only on the first page, is in uppercase and centered over the text. The format of this page should be the same as for the first page of a chapter. Each page of the acknowledgments is numbered in lowercase roman numerals centered beneath the text.

LIST OF ABBREVIATIONS

1.27 A list of abbreviations is desirable only if the writer has devised new abbreviations instead of using commonly accepted ones, such as standard abbreviations of titles of professional journals. A list of abbreviations should be arranged alphabetically by the abbreviation itself, not the spelled-out term. Under the centered generic heading in uppercase, list abbreviations on the left in alphabetical order and leave two to four spaces between the longest abbreviation and its spelled-out term. Align the first letter of all other spelled-out terms and any runover lines with the first letter of the term following the *longest* abbreviation, and use the longest line in the column to center the list on the page(s). Double-space between items, single-space within, as in sample 14.32. A list of abbreviations helps the reader who looks at only a portion of the paper instead of reading it from beginning to end. Even when a paper includes a list of abbreviations, the spelled-out version should be given the first time a term appears, followed by the abbreviation in parentheses.

GLOSSARY

1.28 A paper that contains many foreign words or technical terms and phrases likely to be unfamiliar to the reader should include a list of these, followed by their translations or definitions. The terms should be arranged alphabetically, each typed flush left and followed by a period, a dash, or a colon. The translation or definition follows, with its first word capitalized and ending with a period, unless all definitions consist only of single words or phrases, in which case no final punctuation should be used. If a definition extends to more than one line, the runover lines should be indented five spaces from the left margin. Double-space between items, single-space within, as in sample 14.33.

1.29 If there is more than one glossary, each should start on a new page.

1.30 A glossary placed in the back matter rather than in the front matter follows an appendix, if any, and precedes the bibliography or reference list.

EDITORIAL METHOD

1.31 Following the same format as does the preface (see 1.25), a section devoted to editorial method may be included in the preliminaries to explain the writer's editorial practice or to discuss variant texts, particularly if the paper is a scholarly edition. In practice, however, this discussion is usually part of the introduction. Short, uncomplicated remarks about editorial method—such as a note that capitalization and punctuation have been modernized—may be included in the preface or placed in a note after the first quotation from the edited work.

ABSTRACT

1.32 An abstract, which may or may not be required, briefly summarizes the thesis and contents of the paper. Like the title, it may be used by information services to create lists of papers organized by subject matter. Since each department or discipline has its own requirements, consult the thesis adviser or dissertation office regarding the content, style, placement, and format of the abstract.

TEXT

1.33 The body of the paper is usually separated into well-defined divisions, such as parts, chapters, sections, and subsections. The text may also include parenthetical references, footnotes, or superscript numbers keyed to a reference list or to endnotes.

INTRODUCTION

1.34 The text usually begins with an introduction, which may be called chapter 1. If it is short, the writer may prefer to head it simply INTRODUCTION and reserve the more formal generic heading CHAPTER for the longer sections that compose the body of the paper. Whether it is called chapter 1 or not, the introduction is equivalent to the first chapter and is not part of the preliminaries. Thus the first page of the introduction is page 1 (arabic numeral) of the paper.

PART

1.35 If a work is divided into parts, each comprising one or more chapters, each should be preceded by a part-title page. Part-title pages display only the generic heading, the part number, and any part title. Since the introduction is to the *entire* paper, whether it is titled chapter 1 or not, it is not included in part 1. The first part-title page therefore follows rather than precedes the introduction.

CHAPTER

1.36 The body of the paper is divided into chapters, each beginning on a new page. The generic heading CHAPTER is followed by a number, which may be either spelled out (in capitals) or given as a numeral (arabic or uppercase roman). Conventionally, the entire heading is centered. Some writers omit the word CHAPTER and use only numerals—roman or arabic—in sequence before the headings of the main divisions. The form of the chapter numbers should be different from that used for part numbers (e.g., PART II, CHAPTER 4). The title, which describes the content of the chapter, is also in uppercase, centered below the generic heading (see samples 14.34 and 14.36).

SECTION AND SUBSECTION

1.37   In some papers the chapters or their equivalents are divided into sections, which may in turn be divided into subsections, then into sub-subsections, and so on. Such divisions are customarily given titles, called *subheads* or *subheadings,* which are differentiated typographically and designated *first-, second-,* and *third-level* subheads. The principal, or first-level, subdivision should have greater attention value than the lower levels. Centered headings have more attention value than sideheads (beginning at the left margin), and italic, underlining, or boldface type has more than text type. Attention value is also enhanced by leaving some blank space above and below all but run-in subheads. A suggested plan for five levels of subheads follows.

First level: centered heading in boldface, italicized, or underlined, capitalized headline style:

Traditional Controversy between Medieval Church and State

Second level: centered heading in text type, capitalized headline style:

Reappearance of Religious Legalism

Third level: sidehead in boldface, italicized, or underlined, capitalized headline style:

Legalism and the Poets

Fourth level: sidehead in text type, capitalized sentence style:

The gospel as it is related to Jesus

Fifth level: run-in heading at beginning of paragraph in boldface, italicized, or underlined, capitalized sentence style with a period at the end:

> *The gospel legalized in the church.* The gospel
> that the early Christians preached within the pagan
> sects was also a product of their experience.

1.38   If fewer than five levels are required, the style of these levels may be selected in any suitable *descending order.* A page should never end with a subhead. For the layout of subheadings on a page, see samples 14.31 and 14.35.

BACK MATTER, OR REFERENCE MATTER

Appendix

1.39   An appendix, though by no means an essential part of every paper, is a useful device to make available material that is relevant to the text but not suitable for inclusion in it. An appendix is a group of related items. Appendixes, for example, may contain tables too detailed for text presentation, a large group of illustrations, technical notes on method, schedules and forms used in collecting materials, copies of documents not generally available to the reader, case studies too long to put into the text, and sometimes figures or other illustrative materials. When a writer gathers all the paper's illustrations, they are instead included in a group titled ILLUSTRATIONS placed just before the back matter. If some illustrations are placed in the text, however, any that are grouped in the back matter must be put in an appendix.

1.40   All appendixes go at the end of a paper, not at the ends of chapters.

1.41   Materials of different categories should be placed in separate appendixes. When there is more than one appendix, each is given a number or a letter (APPENDIX 1, etc.; APPENDIX ONE, etc.; APPENDIX A, etc.).

1.42   If there is only one appendix, the writer may or may not give it a title, like a chapter or part title. If a paper has more than one appendix, each must bear a descriptive title, which also appears in the table of contents (see 14.20). On the opening page of each appendix the generic heading and the title are both centered and typed in full capitals.

1.43   Whether an appendix should be single-spaced or double-spaced depends on the nature of the material; spacing need not be the same for all the appendixes. Documents and case studies may well be single-spaced, whereas explanations of methods and procedures should be double-spaced like the text.

1.44 When photocopied documents, such as previously published articles, facsimiles of manuscripts, or questionnaires, appear as separate pages in appendixes, a page number should be added to each photocopy, using arabic numerals within brackets in the upper right corner, indicating their sequence within the pagination of the paper. The brackets show that the page number is not part of the original document. The photocopied documents within an appendix may or may not contain original pagination.

1.45 If an appendix contains photocopied material, the photocopies must be of letter quality (see 13.28, 13.37).

ENDNOTES

1.46 Endnotes, which may have the same content as footnotes, are more common in term papers than in theses or dissertations, where footnotes have traditionally been preferred and parenthetical references (see 10.2–19) are now often recommended. In term papers, endnotes are numbered consecutively throughout the paper. In longer works that are divided into chapters, however, endnotes are numbered consecutively from 1 within each chapter. Superscript arabic numerals are used as indicators in text, but full-sized on-line arabic numerals, followed by periods, precede the endnotes themselves (sample 14.38). All endnotes are grouped in the back matter under the generic heading NOTES, with subheads giving the chapter numbers.

BIBLIOGRAPHY OR REFERENCE LIST

1.47 The bibliography or reference list (see chapters 9 and 10) is the last part of the paper (except in those rare instances where a paper carries an index, like a book). Instructions for the layout of these parts are set forth in samples 14.39–42.

2   Abbreviations and Numbers

Abbreviations 2.1
   Use of Periods 2.2
   Social and Professional Titles and Similar Terms 2.3
   Organizations 2.11
   Geographical Names 2.13
   Measure 2.16
   Scholarship 2.18
      Parts of a Work 2.18
      Unpublished Manuscripts 2.19
      Books of the Bible 2.20
      Classical References 2.22
      General Scholarly Abbreviations 2.23
   For Further Reference 2.28
Numbers 2.29
   General Rule 2.29
   Series 2.31
   Initial Numbers 2.32
   Percentages and Decimals 2.36
   Numerals, Symbols, and Abbreviations 2.37
   Fractions 2.39
   Currencies 2.40
      United States Currency 2.40
      British Currency 2.42
      Other Currencies 2.43
   Numbered Parts of Written Works 2.44
   Date and Time 2.49
      Day, Month, and Year 2.49
      Century 2.53
      Decade 2.54
      Month and Day Names 2.55
      Era 2.56

Time of Day 2.57
Numbers and Names 2.58
    Monarchs and the Like 2.58
    Family Names 2.59
    Government Designations 2.60
    Churches, Lodges, and Unions 2.61
    Street Addresses, Highways, and Telephone Numbers 2.63
Scientific Usage 2.64
Commas within Numbers 2.66
Inclusive Numbers 2.67
Plurals of Numbers 2.68
Numbers in Enumerations 2.70
    Enumerations in Text 2.70
    Numbers Beginning a New Line or Paragraph 2.72
    Outlines 2.73

ABBREVIATIONS

2.1   Though the use of abbreviations in formal writing was traditionally limited to a few prescribed circumstances, during the
past few decades abbreviations have been used increasingly in
writing of all kinds. In tabular matter, notes, bibliographies,
illustrations, and lists, abbreviations are normally preferred
and are formed according to a standard list accepted within
any given field. Such forms of address as *Mr., Mrs.,* and *Dr.*
are almost never spelled out. The writer who must form new
abbreviations for a paper should include a list of abbreviations
in the front matter (see 1.27). For guidelines on hyphenating
and dividing abbreviations, see 3.50.

USE OF PERIODS

2.2   The trend is strongly away from the use of periods, especially
in uppercase abbreviations. In the examples that follow, the
periods have been left wherever they have traditionally appeared. Periods may be omitted from many of these examples,
but it is well to use periods after lowercase abbreviations that
spell words (e.g., *in., act., no.*). A period and a space are used
after the initials of personal names (e.g., *E. F. Bowman*). In an
abbreviation with an internal period (e.g., *N. Y., Ph.D., N.Dak.,
U.S.*), however, there should be no space after that period.

SOCIAL AND PROFESSIONAL TITLES AND SIMILAR TERMS

2.3   Most social titles are abbreviated, whether used with the full name or the last name only (note that there is no period after *Mlle* and *Mme*):

```
Mr.       Mrs.      Ms.
M.        MM.       Messrs.
Mlle      Mme       Dr.
```

2.4   The abbreviations *Sr., Jr., III,* and *IV* (for *Senior, Junior, Third,* and *Fourth*) follow a full name and are not used with the family name alone. The terms are never spelled out when part of a name. Though a comma has traditionally preceded *Jr.* and *Sr.* (but not *III* and *IV*), *The Chicago Manual of Style* now recommends omitting commas in all such cases.

```
Rev. Oliver C. Jones Jr. spoke to the group.

Do you know Ralph Smith Jr.'s address?
```

2.5   Abbreviations for scholarly degrees and titles of respect, which follow full names, are set off by two commas when they are given in text.

```
Laura S. Wells, Ph.D., was on the committee.

The Reverend Jesse E. Thorson, S.T.B., was nominated by
the board of trustees.
```

The following list includes many frequently used abbreviations for scholarly degrees and professional and honorary designations:

A.B., Artium Bacclaureus (Bachelor of Arts)
A.M., Artium Magister (Master of Arts)
B.A., Bachelor of Arts
B.D., Bachelor of Divinity
B.F.A., Bachelor of Fine Arts
B.S., Bachelor of Science
D.B., Divinitatis Baccalaureus (Bachelor of Divinity)
D.D., Divinitatis Doctor (Doctor of Divinity)
D.D.S., Doctor of Dental Surgery
D.Min., Doctor of Ministry
D.O., Doctor of Osteopathy
D.V.M., Doctor of Veterinary Medicine
Esq., Esquire

F.A.I.A., Fellow of the American Institute of Architects
F.R.S., Fellow of the Royal Society
J.D., Juris Doctor (Doctor of Law)
J.P., Justice of the Peace
L.H.D., Litterarum Humaniorum Doctor (Doctor of Humanities)
Litt.D., Litterarum Doctor (Doctor of Letters)
LL.B., Legum Baccalaureus (Bachelor of Laws)
LL.D., Legum Doctor (Doctor of Laws)
M.A., Master of Arts
M.B.A., Master of Business Administration
M.D., Medicinae Doctor (Doctor of Medicine)
M.F.A., Master of Fine Arts
M.P., Member of Parliament
M.S., Master of Science
Ph.B., Philosophiae Baccalaureus (Bachelor of Philosophy)
Ph.D., Philosophiae Doctor (Doctor of Philosophy)
Ph.G., Graduate in Pharmacy
S.B., Scientiae Baccalaureus (Bachelor of Science)
S.M., Scientiae Magister (Master of Science)
S.T.B., Sacrae Theologiae Baccalaureus (Bachelor of Sacred Theology)

2.6   Abbreviate *doctor (Dr.)* before a name, but spell it out when it is not followed by a name:

Dr. Shapiro brought about a total recovery.

The doctor was an expert in her field.

2.7   Spell out a civil, military, professional, or religious title when it precedes the family name alone:

Senator Proxmire   General Patton

But use the appropriate abbreviation before a full name:

Sen. William F. Proxmire   Gen. George S. Patton

2.8   Spell out *Reverend, Honorable,* and *Colonel* if preceded by *the;* otherwise abbreviate to *Rev., Hon.,* or *Col.* Never use these titles, either spelled out or abbreviated, with family names alone. Use them only when the title is followed by the person's full name or by *Mr., Mrs., Miss, Ms.,* or *Dr.* with the family name alone, as may be appropriate:

Col. Arthur Charles reviewed the procedures.

The ceremony was in honor of the Reverend Martin Luther King Jr.'s birthday observance.

```
Rev. Dr. Wilson gave the address.
```
```
The Honorable Mr. Collins closed the final session of
the conference.
```

Never use:

```
Rev. Bentley
Reverend Bentley
the Rev. Bentley
the Reverend Bentley
```

2.9   *Saint* may be abbreviated when it stands before the name of a Christian saint:

```
St. Thomas Aquinas      SS. Augustine and Benedict
```

But *Saint* is omitted before the names of apostles, evangelists, and church fathers:

```
Matthew      Mark         Luke         Peter
Paul         Augustine    Ambrose      Jerome
```

2.10   When *Saint* forms part of a personal name, the bearer's usage is followed:

```
Etienne Geoffroy Saint-Hilaire
Charles-Camille Saint-Saëns
Muriel St. Clare Byrne
Ruth St. Denis
```

ORGANIZATIONS

2.11   The names of government agencies, network broadcasting companies, associations, fraternal and service organizations, unions, and other groups are often abbreviated, even in text, preferably after one spelled-out use. Such abbreviations are in full capitals with no periods:

```
AAAS     AFL-CIO     AMA     AT&T       FTC      HOLC
NAACP    NAFTA       NBC     NFL        NIMH     NSF
OPEC     TVA         UN      UNESCO     VA       YMCA
```

2.12   Within the text, company names should be given in their full form, without including the terms *Inc.* or *Ltd.* and without capitalizing the word *the,* even when it is part of a company's full name:

```
A. G. Becker and Company was incorporated in 1894.
```
```
The book was published by the University of Chicago
Press.
```

In notes, bibliographies, parenthetical references, reference lists, and the like, the following abbreviations may be freely (but consistently) used:

```
Bro.    Bros.    Co.    Corp.    Inc.    Ltd.    &
```

GEOGRAPHICAL NAMES

2.13 Within the text, spell out the names of countries, states, counties, provinces, territories, bodies of water, mountains, and the like, with the exception of the former Union of Soviet Socialist Republics, commonly referred to as the USSR. In lists, tabular matter, notes, bibliographies, and indexes, the following abbreviations for state names may be used (the two-letter form for mailing addresses is often useful in other contexts as well):

Ala.	AL	Kans.	KS	Ohio	OH
Alaska	AK	Ky.	KY	Okla.	OK
Amer.Samoa	AS	La.	LA	Oreg. *or* Ore.	OR
Ariz.	AZ	Maine	ME	Pa.	PA
Ark.	AR	Md.	MD	P.R.	PR
Calif.	CA	Mass.	MA	R.I.	RI
C.Z.	CZ	Mich.	MI	S.C.	SC
Colo.	CO	Minn.	MN	S.Dak.	SD
Conn.	CT	Miss.	MS	Tenn.	TN
Del.	DE	Mo.	MO	Tex.	TX
D.C.	DC	Mont.	MT	Utah	UT
Fla.	FL	Nebr.	NE	Vt.	VT
Ga.	GA	Nev.	NV	Va.	VA
Guam	GU	N.H.	NH	V.I.	VI
Hawaii	HI	N.J.	NJ	Wash.	WA
Idaho	ID	N.Mex.	NM	W.Va.	WV
Ill.	IL	N.Y.	NY	Wis. *or* Wisc.	WI
Ind.	IN	N.C.	NC	Wyo.	WY
Iowa	IA	N.Dak.	ND		

2.14 Spell out the prefixes of most geographical names (e.g., *Fort Wayne, South Orange, Port Arthur*) within the text. *Saint* may be shortened to *St.,* but it must then be abbreviated consistently:

```
Mount St. Helens has erupted several times.

From northeast Paris it is less than an hour to Saint-
Cloud on the Métro.
```

2.15   Within the text, spell out all the following words. In close-set matter, the abbreviations may be used:

Avenue	Ave.	Street	St.
Boulevard	Blvd.	Terrace	Terr.
Building	Bldg.	North	N.
Court	Ct.	South	S.
Drive	Dr.	East	E.
Expressway	Expy.	West	W.
Lane	La. *or* Ln.	Northeast	NE
Parkway	Pkwy.	Northwest	NW
Place	Pl.	Southeast	SE
Road	Rd.	Southwest	SW
Square	Sq.		

But always use the abbreviations *NW, NE, SE,* and *SW* where they follow street names in city addresses:

```
Lake Shore Drive is safer than the Dan Ryan Expressway,
where there is truck traffic.

He spent several years in Southeast Asia.

The shop is at 245 Seventeenth Street NW.
```

MEASURE

2.16   In nontechnical writing, spell out expressions of dimension, distance, volume, weight, degree, and so on:

```
five miles     150 pounds     14.5 meters
```

2.17   In scientific and technical writing, standard abbreviations for units of measure are used if the amount is given in numerals. Most guides to scientific and technical writing (several are included in the bibliography) list standard abbreviations acceptable within a given discipline. For a general introduction to the use of abbreviations for units of measure, consult *The Chicago Manual of Style,* fourteenth edition, 14.36–53. A full explanation of the International System of Units (*Système international d'unités,* abbreviated *SI*) appears in *General Principles concerning Quantities, Units, and Symbols,* compiled by the International Standards Organization (ISO) and published in Geneva in 1981.

SCHOLARSHIP

PARTS OF A WORK

2.18 Spell out and do not capitalize (unless in a heading or at the beginning of a sentence) the words *book, chapter, part, volume, section, scene, verse, column, page, figure, plate,* and so on, except when such a term is followed by a number in a note or parenthetical reference, in which case the following abbreviations should be used: *bk., chap., pt., vol., sect., sc., v. (vv.), coll., p. (pp.), fig., pt.* Add *s* for the plural unless otherwise shown. Chapter numbers in text references are given in arabic numerals, even when the actual chapter numbers are spelled out or in roman numerals. The words *act, line,* and *table* should never be abbreviated.

UNPUBLISHED MANUSCRIPTS

2.19 When referring to unpublished manuscripts, spell out the terms used to describe them within the text, but in notes, bibliographies, and reference lists, use the abbreviations listed below. Terms not in this list should always be spelled out. The abbreviations are used by many curators and librarians. See 8.131–32, 11.49–50, and 11.52–55 for examples of notes and reference list entries using abbreviations listed here or using spelled-out forms, as needed.

Letter	L
Letter signed	LS
Autograph letter signed	ALS
Typewritten letter	TL
Typewritten letter signed	TLS
Document	D
Document signed	DS
Autograph document	AD
Autograph document signed	ADS
Typewritten document	TD
Typewritten document signed	TDS
Autograph manuscript	AMs
Autograph manuscript signed	AMsS
Typewritten manuscript	TMs
Typewritten manuscript signed	TMsS
Card	C

Autograph card	AC
Autograph card signed	ACS
Typewritten card	TC
Typewritten card signed	TCS
Autograph note	AN
Autograph note signed	ANS

This list is reprinted, with minor changes, from *Modern Manuscripts: A Practical Manual for Their Management, Care, and Use,* by Kenneth W. Duckett (Nashville: American Association for State and Local History, 1975), 143–44, by permission of the publisher. © 1975 by the American Association for State and Local History.

BOOKS OF THE BIBLE

2.20   When referring to whole chapters or to whole books of the Bible or the Apocrypha, spell out the names of the books (do not italicize or underline them):

```
Jeremiah, chapters 42-44, records the flight of the
Jews to Egypt when Jerusalem fell in 586 B.C.

The Revelation of St. John the Divine, known as
"Revelation," closes the New Testament.
```

2.21   When scriptural passages are cited by verse in a paper, whether in text, parenthetical references, or notes, abbreviate the names of the books, using arabic numerals if they are numbered; write the chapter and verse numbers in arabic numerals with either a colon or a period between them; and follow the chapter and verse numbers with the abbreviation for the version of the Bible or Apocrypha from which the passage was taken.

```
1 Song of Sol. 2.1-5 RSV     Ru 3:14 NAB
```

For standard biblical abbreviations, see *The Chicago Manual of Style,* fourteenth edition, 14.34–35.

CLASSICAL REFERENCES

2.22   In a paper containing many classical references, both the name of the author and the title of the work may be abbreviated after they have been spelled out in full when cited the first time,

whether in text or notes. Often the names of well-known periodicals and reference tools are also abbreviated after being
spelled out in the first citation. The most widely accepted standard for such abbreviations is the comprehensive list in the
front of the *Oxford Classical Dictionary.*

```
Thucydides History of the Peloponnesian War 2.40.2-3
Thud. 2.40.2-3
Homer Odyssey 9.266-71
Hom. Od. 9.266-71
```

GENERAL SCHOLARLY ABBREVIATIONS

2.23   General abbreviations such as *etc., e.g.,* and *i.e.* should be confined to parenthetical references within the text. The abbreviations *ibid., cf.,* and *s.v.* are preferably used only in notes and
other scholarly apparatus.

2.24   An abbreviation begins with a capital when it is the first word
of a note and whenever the usual rules for capitalization apply.

2.25   The word *sic* is italicized or underlined, but not most other
Latin words or abbreviations commonly used in footnotes, bibliographies, tabular matter, and so on (see 2.26). See also 5.36.

2.26   The following abbreviations and Latin words are commonly
used in scholarly text. Add *s* for the plural unless otherwise
shown.

     act., active
     app., appendix
     art., article
     b., born
     bk., book
     c., copyright
     ca., *circa*, about, approximately
     cf., *confer,* compare (Note that *confer* is the Latin word for
        "compare"; *cf.* must not be used as the abbreviation for
        the English "confer," nor should it be used to mean "see.")
     ch., chapter (in law references)
     chap., chapter
     col., column
     comp., compiler; compiled by
     d., died

dept., department

div., division

ed., editor; edition; edited by

e.g., *exempli gratia,* for example

et al., *et alia,* and others

etc., *et cetera,* and so forth

et seq., *et sequentes,* and the following

fig., figure

fl., *floruit,* flourished (for use when birth and death dates are not known)

ibid., *ibidem,* in the same place

id., *idem,* the same (used to refer to persons, except in law citations; not to be confused with ibid.)

i.e., *id est,* that is

infra, below

l. (el), line (*plural,* ll.) (Not recommended because the abbreviation in the singular might be mistaken for "one" and the plural for "eleven.")

n., note, footnote (*plural,* nn.)

n.d., no date

no., number

n.p., no place; no publisher

n.s., new series

o.s., old series

p., page (*plural,* pp.)

par., paragraph

passim, here and there

pt., part

q.v., *quod vide,* which see (for use with cross-references)

sc., scene

sec., section

sic, so, thus

supp. or suppl., supplement

supra, above

s.v., *sub verbo, sub voce,* under the word (*plural,* s.vv.; used in references to encyclopedias and dictionaries)

trans., translator; translated by

v., verse (*plural,* vv.)

viz., *videlicet,* namely

vol., volume

vs., *versus,* against (v. in law references)

2.27   In quoting from constitutions, bylaws, and the like within the text, the words *section* and *article* are spelled out the first time they are used and abbreviated thereafter, traditionally in uppercase, and arabic numerals are used:

```
SECTION 1. The name of the . . .
SEC. 2. The object of the . . .
ARTICLE 235. It shall be the . . .
ART. 235. It shall be the duty . . .
```

References in running text should be spelled out in lowercase:

```
In article 256 it is specified that . . .
```

Standard abbreviations used by many law reviews appear in *A Uniform System of Citation,* fifteenth edition (1991).

FOR FURTHER REFERENCE

2.28   *Merriam-Webster's Collegiate Dictionary* includes a great many abbreviations from all fields, arranged in letter-by-letter alphabetical order. To identify a rare or unfamiliar abbreviation, consult the *Reverse Acronyms, Initialisms, and Abbreviations Dictionary,* 17th ed., 3 vols. (Detroit: Gale Research Company, 1992–94), available at most libraries.

NUMBERS

GENERAL RULE

2.29   In scientific and statistical material, all numbers are expressed in numerals. In nonscientific material, numbers are sometimes spelled out and sometimes expressed in numerals, according to prescribed conventions. The general rule followed by many writers and by the University of Chicago Press is to spell out all numbers through one hundred and any of the whole numbers followed by *hundred, thousand, hundred thousand, million,* and so on. For all other numbers, numerals are used.

```
At that time the combined population of the three
districts was less than four million.
```

```
There are 514 seniors in the graduating class.
```

2.30 The general rule applies to ordinal as well as cardinal numbers:

    On the 122d and 123d days of his recovery, he received
    his eighteenth and nineteenth letters from home.

Note that the preferred numeral form of the ordinals *second* and *third* adds *d* alone *(2d, 3d)*, not *nd* and *rd (2nd, 3rd)*.

SERIES

2.31 The general rule must be modified when numbers above *and* below one hundred appear in a series, or group, applying to the same kind of thing. Here all are expressed in numerals:

    Of the group surveyed, 186 students had studied French,
    142 had studied Spanish, and 36 had studied Latin for
    three years or more.

INITIAL NUMBERS

2.32 A sentence should never begin with a numeral, even when there are numerals in the rest of the sentence. Either spell out the first number or recast the sentence:

    Two hundred and fifty passengers escaped injury; 175
    sustained minor injuries; 110 were so seriously hurt
    that they required hospitalization.

>   *or better*

    Of the passengers, 250 escaped injury, 175 sustained
    minor injuries, and 110 required hospitalization.

2.33 To avoid confusion, you may spell out one set of numbers in an expression that involves two or more series:

    In a test given six months later, 14 children made no
    errors; 64 made one to two errors; 97 made three to
    four errors.

2.34 Although a round number occurring in isolation is spelled out (see 2.29), several round numbers close together are expressed in numerals:

    They shipped 1,500 books in the first order, 8,000 in
    the second, and 100,000 in the third; all together
    there were now about 1,000,000 volumes in the
    warehouse.

2.35 Very large round numbers are frequently expressed in numerals and units of millions or billions:

> This means that welfare programs will require about $7.8 million per day, compared with $3.2 million spent each day at the current rate of inflation.

PERCENTAGES AND DECIMALS

2.36 Numerals should be used to express decimal fractions and percentages. The word *percent* should be written out except in scientific and statistical writing, where the symbol % may be used:

> With interest at 8 percent, the monthly payment would amount to $12.88, which he noted was exactly 2.425 times the amount he was accustomed to put in savings monthly.

> Grades of 3.8 and 95% are equivalent.

When fractional and whole numbers are used in the same sentence or paragraph, both should be expressed as numerals (see also 2.40):

> The average number of children born to college graduates dropped from 2.4 to 2 per couple.

In scientific contexts decimal fractions of less than 1.00 begin with a zero if the quantity expressed is capable of equaling or exceeding 1.00:

> a mean of 0.73   the ratio 0.85

NUMERALS, SYMBOLS, AND ABBREVIATIONS

2.37 Use the symbol for *percent* (%) only when it is preceded by a number. Note that *percentage,* not *percent* or %, is the correct expression when no number is given:

> The September scores for students enrolled in summer school showed an improvement of 70.1% [or 70.1 percent] over test scores recorded in June. Thus the percentage of achievers in the second test indicated that summer school had resulted in higher scores in a majority of cases.

2.38 The number preceding either *percent* or % is never spelled out (except when beginning a sentence):

> 15 percent   55%

FRACTIONS

2.39   A fraction standing alone should be spelled out, but a unit composed of a whole number and a fraction should be expressed in numerals:

Trade and commodity services accounted for nine-tenths
of all international receipts and payments.

Cabinets with 10¹/₂-by-32¹/₄-inch shelves were
installed.

CURRENCIES

UNITED STATES CURRENCY

2.40   The general rule (see 2.29) applies in isolated references to amounts of money in United States currency. If the amount is spelled out, so are the words *dollars* and *cents;* if numerals are used, the dollar sign ($) precedes them:

Rarely do they spend more than five dollars a week on
recreation.

The report showed $135 collected in fines.

Fractional amounts of money over one dollar appear in numerals, as do other decimal fractions ($1.75). When both fractional amounts and whole-dollar amounts are used in the same sentence (and only then), the whole-dollar amounts are shown with a decimal point and zeros:

The same article is sold by some stores for $1.75, by
others for $1.95, and by still others for $2.00

2.41   The expression of very large amounts of money, which may be cumbersome whether spelled out or written in numerals, should follow the rule for large round numbers (see 2.35), using units of millions or billions with numerals preceded by the dollar sign:

Japan's exports to Taiwan, which averaged $60 million
between 1954 and 1958, rose sharply to $210 million in
1965 and $250 million in 1966.

The deficit that year was $120.4 billion.

2.42   British currency is expressed in pounds and pence, very like dollars and cents:

```
two pounds              twenty-five pence
£3.50                   55 p.
```

Before decimalization in 1971, British currency was expressed in pounds, shillings, and pence:

```
two shillings and sixpence
£12 17s. 6d.
```

or

```
£12.17.6
```

The term *billion* should not be used for British sums, since *billion* in British terms equals *trillion* in United States terminology.

2.43   Most currencies follow a system like that of the United States, employing unit symbols before the numerals. They do vary, however, in their expression of large numbers and decimals. For papers that deal with sums in currencies other than those of the United States or Great Britain, consult the table "Foreign Money" in the U.S. Government Printing Office *Style Manual* (1984).

NUMBERED PARTS OF WRITTEN WORKS

2.44   With few exceptions (see 8.70, 8.126, and 12.25), all the numbered parts of printed works are cited in arabic numerals. A reference to preliminary pages numbered with lowercase roman numerals, however, should also employ that style.

2.45   Citations to public documents and unpublished manuscript material should use exactly the kind of numerals found in the source.

2.46   In biblical, classical, and many medieval references in text as well as in notes, bibliographies, and reference lists, the different levels of division of a work (book, section, line, etc.) are given in arabic numerals and separated by periods (no spaces precede or follow these periods). Note that in biblical references either a colon or a period is acceptable:

```
Heb. 13:3
2 Kings 11.12
Ovid Amores 1.7.27
Augustine De civitate Dei 20.2
```

In a paper, commas are used between several references to the same level, and a hyphen is used between inclusive numbers:

```
1 Thess. 4:1, 5
Gen. 25.19-37
Cicero De officiis 1.33, 140
```

2.47 Fragments of classical and biblical texts (some only recently discovered) are often not uniformly numbered or may have no numbering whatever. The same is true of some modern manuscripts. In citing such materials, indicate any ordering of pages that has been added, whether by an individual or an institution holding the collection, by setting added numbering in the exact style in which it is written on the original manuscript (letters, arabic or roman numerals, uppercase or lower case, subscript or superscript, etc.) and enclosing this notation in brackets. Put a space after the final bracket, then give the full name of the person or institution that ordered the text. In subsequent references this name may be abbreviated.

2.48 If unpaginated fragments or manuscripts are published in collections, the numbering of the material will be unique to a particular edition. In citing published fragments and other documents unpaginated in the original, do not use brackets around the numbers imposed by an editor or institution. Instead, the first time a collection is referred to, give the editor's name immediately after the fragment number. In subsequent references, use only initials:

```
Empedocles frag. 115 Diels-Kranz
Hesiod frag. 239.1 Merkebach and West
Empedocles frag. 111 D.
Hesiod frag. 220 M.-W.
```

DATE AND TIME

DAY, MONTH, AND YEAR

2.49 One of the two permissible styles for expressing day, month, and year should be followed consistently throughout a paper. The first, which omits punctuation, is preferred:

```
On 28 June 1970 the convocation Pacem in Maribus was
held.
```

If the alternative sequence month-day-year is used, the year is set off by commas:

```
On June 28, 1970, the convocation Pacem in Maribus was
held.
```

2.50 Note that when the day, month, and year are mentioned as in the foregoing examples, *st, d,* or *th* does not appear after the day. When the day alone is given, without the month or the year, or when the number of the day is separated from the name of the month by one or more words, the preferred style is to spell out the day:

```
The sequence of events of 10 June is unclear.

The sequence of events of the eleventh of June is
unclear.

The date set was the twenty-ninth.
```

2.51 When month and year alone are mentioned, omit punctuation between them:

```
She graduated in December 1985.
```

2.52 In formal writing, references to the year should not be abbreviated (e.g., '95).

CENTURY

2.53 References to particular centuries should be spelled out, in lowercase. Hyphenate such references only when they serve as adjectives, as in the first and fifth examples below. See also 4.7.

```
seventeenth-century literature
the eighteenth century
the twenty-first century
```

```
the mid-twentieth century
late sixteenth-century ideas
```

DECADE

2.54   References to decades take two forms. The context sometimes determines the one chosen:

```
The 1890s saw an enormous increase in the use of
manufactured gas.

During the thirties, traffic decreased by 50 percent.
```

MONTH AND DAY NAMES

2.55   Spell out the names of months and of days when they occur in text, whether alone or in dates. In notes, bibliographies, tables, and other closely set matter, the following designations are permissible if used consistently: Jan., Feb., Mar., Apr., May, June, July, Aug., Sept., Oct., Nov., Dec.; Sun., Mon., Tues., Wed., Thurs., Fri., Sat.

ERA

2.56   For era designations use the abbreviations B.C., A.D., B.C.E., C.E. ("before Christ," *anno Domini,* "before the common era," "of the common era"), in capitals. A.D. precedes the year number; the other designations follow it.

```
Solomon's Temple was destroyed by the Babylonians in
586 B.C. Rebuilt in 515 B.C., it was destroyed by the
Romans in A.D. 70.
```

TIME OF DAY

2.57   Except when A.M. or P.M. is used, time of day should be spelled out in text matter. Never add *in the morning* after A.M. or *in the evening* after P.M., and never use *o'clock* with either A.M. or P.M. or with numerals:

```
The train was scheduled to arrive at 7:10 A.M.

The meeting was called for 8:00 P.M.

The meeting was called for eight o'clock in the
evening.
```

Where the context makes it clear whether morning or evening is meant, these terms need not be expressed.

```
The breakfast meeting was set for eight o'clock.
```

```
The night operator takes calls from eleven to seven.
```

Midnight is written as 12:00 P.M., noon as 12:00 M. ("meridian").

NUMBERS AND NAMES

MONARCHS AND THE LIKE

2.58   Emperors, sovereigns, or popes with the same name are differentiated by numerals, traditionally capital roman numerals:

```
Charles V        Henry VIII      Elizabeth II
Napoleon III     Louis XIV       John XXIII
```

FAMILY NAMES

2.59   Male family members with identical names are sometimes differentiated in the same way as monarchs:

```
Adlai E. Stevenson III
```

See also 2.4.

GOVERNMENT DESIGNATIONS

2.60   Particular dynasties, governments, governing bodies, political divisions, and military subdivisions are commonly designated by an ordinal number before the noun. Numbers through one hundred should be spelled out and capitalized; those over one hundred, written in numerals:

```
Nineteenth Dynasty
Eighty-first Congress
107th Congress
Fifth Republic
First Continental Congress
Third Reich
Eleventh Ward
```

CHURCHES, LODGES, AND UNIONS

2.61   Numbers before the names of churches or religious organizations should be spelled out in ordinal form and capitalized:

> Eighteenth Church of Christ, Scientist
> Seventh-Day Adventists

2.62   Local branches of fraternal lodges and of unions bear numbers that should be expressed in arabic numerals following the name:

> Typographical Union no. 16
>
> American Legion, Department of California, Leon Robert Post no. 1248

STREET ADDRESSES, HIGHWAYS, AND TELEPHONE NUMBERS

2.63   It is preferable to spell out the names of numbered streets through one hundred for appearance and ease of reading, but street (as well as building) addresses, highway numbers, and telephone numbers should be expressed in numerals:

> The address is 500 East Fifty-eighth Street, Chicago, Illinois 60637. The telephone number is (312) 321-6530.
>
> The meeting took place at 1040 First National Bank Building.
>
> The state will have to repave California 17, Interstate 80, and Route 30 [or U.S. 30].

SCIENTIFIC USAGE

2.64   Scientific papers call for numbers and numerical units of measurement, making numerals, symbols, and abbreviations more common in scientific writing than in nonscientific writing. Aside from a few rules set down here, the writer must settle on the scheme to use—preferably when working on the first draft—and maintain the same usage throughout the paper.

2.65   In mathematical text, the demands for the use of symbols and abbreviations, particularly in equations, are so complicated and vary so much from one paper to another that no suggestions can be given here. Students in this field should receive training in correct usage as part of their study of the science.

Editors of some mathematical periodicals have prepared manuals for writers, which give useful suggestions (see the bibliography). See also the chapter "Mathematics in Type" in *The Chicago Manual of Style,* fourteenth edition. For a brief discussion of equations and formulas in papers prepared on computer systems, see 13.18 in this manual.

COMMAS WITHIN NUMBERS

2.66 For the most part, in numbers of one thousand or more, the thousands are marked off with commas:

    1,500   12,275,500   1,475,525,000

No comma is used, however, in page numbers, street addresses, telephone numbers, zip codes, four-digit year numbers, decimal fractions of less than one, and chapter numbers of fraternal organizations and the like:

    The bibliography is on pages 1012-20.

    In the coastal district the peel thickness plus the
    pulp diameter of the Eureka lemon was 0.1911 for fruit
    from the top of the tree and 0.2016 for fruit from the
    bottom.

    The Leon Robert Post no. 1248 was established in 1946.

Note, however, that in year dates of more than four figures, the comma is employed:

    10,000 B.C.

INCLUSIVE NUMBERS

2.67 The term *inclusive numbers* (or *continued numbers*) refers to the first and last number of a numerical sequence, such as page numbers or years. Inclusive numbers in a paper are separated by a hyphen and either given in full (1978–1979) or expressed according to the following scheme, taken from *The Chicago Manual of Style,* fourteenth edition, 8.69.

FIRST NUMBER	SECOND NUMBER	EXAMPLES
Less than 100	Use all digits	3–10, 71–72, 96–117

100 or multiple of 100	Use all digits	100–104, 600–613, 1100–1123
101 through 109 (in multiples of 100)	Use changed part only, omitting unneeded zeros	107–8, 505–17, 1002–6
110 through 199 (in multiples of 100)	Use two digits, or more if needed	321–25, 415–532, 1536–38, 1496–504, 14325–28, 11564–78, 13792–803

The fourteenth edition of the *Chicago Manual* offers a simpler alternative system for inclusive numbers in which the second number includes only the changed part of the first (8.70):

3–10	600–13	1002–6	1496–504
71–2	100–23	321–5	14325–8
96–117	107–8	415–532	11564–78
100–4	505–17	1536–42	13729–803

The principal uses of the foregoing scheme are for page numbers and other numbered parts of written works and for inclusive year dates:

```
These cities were discussed on pages 2-14, 45-46, 125-
26, 200-210, 308-9.
```

```
He lost everything he owned in the years 1933-36 of the
Great Depression.
```

```
This chapter covers the Napoleonic victories of 1800-
1801.
```

PLURALS OF NUMBERS

2.68 Plurals of numbers expressed in numerals are formed by adding *s* alone (not apostrophe and *s*):

```
Many K-70s were being driven on West German roads in
the 1970s.
```

```
Pilots of 747s undergo special training.
```

```
There was a heavy demand to trade 6½s for the new
8¼s.
```

2.69 Plurals of spelled-out numbers are formed like the plurals of other nouns:

```
There were many more twelves and fourteens on sale than
thirty-twos, thirty-fours, and thirty-sixes.
```

```
Most of the women were in their thirties or forties.
```

Numbers in Enumerations

ENUMERATIONS IN TEXT

2.70 Numbers (or letters) used to enumerate items in text stand out better when in parentheses:

```
He gave two reasons for his resignation: (1) advancing
age and (2) gradually failing eyesight.
```

2.71 When enumerated items appear in text that cites items in a reference list by number (see 10.33), use italic or underlined letters in parentheses for the enumeration rather than arabic numerals:

```
Haskin's latest theory (2) has several drawbacks: (a)
it is not based on current evidence, (b) it has no
clinical basis, and (c) it has a weak theoretical
grounding.
```

NUMBERS BEGINNING A NEW LINE OR PARAGRAPH

2.72 When each numbered item in an enumeration without subdivisions starts on a new line, they most often begin with arabic numerals followed by a period. The items may be given paragraph indention with the runover lines starting at the margin:

```
    1. The nature of the relationship between library
quality and library use.
```

Or the numbers may be flush with the margin, with runover lines aligned with the first line of substantive matter.

```
 9. Selective initial dissemination of published
    material--a direct responsibility of the library
10. Arrangement and organization of the library
```

In both styles, the periods after the numerals must be aligned. Periods are omitted at the ends of items unless the items constitute complete sentences or whole paragraphs (see 3.57).

OUTLINES

2.73   For an outline or other enumeration with subdivisions, the following scheme of notation and indention is recommended. It is not necessary to use a capital roman numeral for the first level when there are fewer divisions than shown in the example. The first level may well begin with A or with arabic 1:

```
    I.  Wars of the nineteenth century
        A.  United States
            1.  Civil War, 1861-65
                a)  Cause
                    (1)  Slavery
                        (a)  Compromise
                            i)  Missouri Compromise
                            ii)  Compromise of 1850 . . .
                b)  Result
    .  .  .  .  .  .  .  .  .  .  .  .  .  .  .  .  .  .  .  .  .
   II.  Wars of the twentieth century
        A.  United States
            1.  First World War . . . . . . . . . . . .
```

Headings should be capitalized sentence style (see 4.9).

3   Spelling and Punctuation

Spelling 3.1
    Plurals 3.2
        Proper Names 3.2
        Capital Letters 3.5
        Letters and Abbreviations 3.6
    Possessives 3.7
    Plurals and Possessives of Compounds 3.11
    Compound Words 3.12
    Division of Words 3.35
        General Rules 3.35
        Special Rules 3.42
Punctuation 3.54
    Period 3.55
    Question Mark 3.60
    Exclamation Point 3.63
    Comma 3.65
    Semicolon 3.84
    Colon 3.88
    Dash 3.91
    Parentheses 3.98
    Brackets 3.99
    Other Punctuation Marks 3.101
    Multiple Punctuation 3.103
    A Warning for Computer Users 3.111

SPELLING

3.1   Spelling in a paper should agree with the best American usage and must be consistent—except, of course, in quotations, where the original must be followed exactly. The authority recommended for spelling and for syllabication (division of words at the ends of lines) is *Webster's Third New International Dictionary* or its most recent abridgment (currently, *Merriam-Webster's Collegiate Dictionary,* tenth edition), using the first spelling where there is a choice. The spelling of many biographical and geographical names is listed at the back of *Webster's Collegiate Dictionary.* For further reference consult *Webster's New Biographical Dictionary* and *Webster's New Geographical Dictionary.*

PLURALS

PROPER NAMES

3.2 Plurals of the names of persons and of other proper nouns are formed by adding *s* or *es* without changing a final *y* to *ie* as required for common nouns.

3.3 Add *s* to all names except those ending in *s, x,* or *z,* or in *ch* or *sh:*

the Andersons	the Costellos	the Frys
the Bradleys	the Joyces	the Pettees

3.4 Add *es* to names ending in *s, x,* or *z,* or in *ch* or *sh:*

the Rosses	the Coxes	the Marshes
the Jenkinses	the Rodriguezes	the Finches

CAPITAL LETTERS

3.5 Form the plurals of most single and multiple capital letters used as nouns by adding *s* alone:

The three Rs are taught at the two YMCAs.

LETTERS AND ABBREVIATIONS

3.6 The plurals of letters, whether lowercase or capital, are often formed with an apostrophe and a roman *s,* but if the letter is italic or underlined the plural may be formed by adding a roman *s* without the apostrophe. Either style, of course, must be used consistently.

All the examples were labeled by letter; the *a*'s were tested first, the *b*'s second, and so on.

```
The A's, I's, and S's in the directory were checked by
   _         _        _
one group.
```

or

```
   . . . ; the as were tested first, the bs second, and
so on.

   . . . ; the as were tested first, the bs second, and
            __                  __
so on.

The As, Is, and Ss . . .

The As, Is, and Ss . . .
    _   _        __
```

The plurals of uppercase abbreviations with internal periods are formed by adding an apostrophe and roman *s:*

```
The B.A.'s and B.S.'s conferred were almost ten times
the number of M.A.'s, M.S.'s, and Ph.D.'s.
```

Noun abbreviations with a single terminal period usually form their plurals by adding *s* before the period:

```
We used 6 lbs. of pressure.
The patient was 45 yrs. old.
```

POSSESSIVES

3.7   Form the possessive of a proper name in the singular by adding an apostrophe and *s:*

```
        Jones's book       Marx's ideology
        Stevens's poems    Diaz's revolt
        Kinross's farm     Finch's candidacy
```

But see the exceptions noted below (3.8–9).

3.8   The possessive of the names Jesus and Moses is traditionally formed by adding an apostrophe alone:

```
        in Jesus' name    Moses' leadership
```

Names of more than one syllable with an unaccented ending pronounced *eez* are also exceptions based on euphony. Many Greek and hellenized names fit this pattern:

```
        Aristophanes' plays       Xerxes' victories
        Charles Yerkes' ideas     R. S. Surtees' novels
```

3.9   For some common nouns as well, euphony dictates adding only an apostrophe:

```
for conscience' sake
for appearance' sake
for righteousness' sake
```

3.10   Form the possessive of a plural proper name (the Bradleys, the Costellos, etc.) by adding an apostrophe to the accepted plural (see 3.3–4):

```
the Bradleys' house        the Rodriguezes' mine
the Costellos' ranch       the Finches' yacht
```

PLURALS AND POSSESSIVES OF COMPOUNDS

3.11   The plurals of prepositional-phrase compounds follow the rule governing the first noun of the compound:

```
brothers-in-law     commanders-in-chief     men-of-war
```

The possessives of the same compound words are formed as follows:

```
my brother-in-law's business
the commander-in-chief's dispatches
the man-of-war's launching
```

COMPOUND WORDS

3.12   The hyphen is used in many compound words, but the trend now is away from the use, or overuse, of hyphens. Which compound words should be hyphenated, which left open, and which spelled as one word is a difficult question. The unabridged Webster's dictionary gives the answer for most noun forms and for many adjective forms. Nevertheless, some are not included. Principles of hyphenation for some of these are given in the following paragraphs.

3.13   Relationship compounds are either closed, hyphenated, or open. Compounds with *grand* are closed; those with *great* are hyphenated; and the rest are open:

```
grandmother            parent organization
great-grandmother      father figure
```

3.14 Compounds made up of two nouns representing different but equal functions are hyphenated:

```
author-critic          artist-inventor
composer-director      architect-painter
city-state             scholar-poet
```

3.15 Compounds made up of two nouns expressing a single function are either open or closed.

```
information technologies    policymaker
dissertation adviser        jobholder
```

3.16 Compounds spelled as one word may be found in most unabridged dictionaries; if not listed, the compound should be open.

```
dogcatcher     bookkeeper     bathtub
```

3.17 Compounds ending with *elect* should be hyphenated except when the name of the office is two or more words:

```
president-elect
```

but

```
county clerk elect
```

3.18 Most compounds describing a person's character are hyphenated, but some are open:

```
stay-at-home         flash in the pan
stick-in-the-mud     ball of fire
```

3.19 The numerator and denominator of a spelled-out fractional number should be separated by a hyphen unless either already contains a hyphen:

```
two-thirds          one-half
```

but

```
one thirty-second    sixty-five hundredths
```

3.20 Many compounds ending with *book* have been accepted into the general English vocabulary as single words and are spelled so in Webster; others are treated as two words:

```
checkbook           textbook
```

but

```
telephone book    pattern book
```

3.21 The same applies to compounds ending in *house:*

clubhouse   greenhouse

but

business house   rest house

3.22 Spell as separate words adjective forms composed of an adverb ending in *ly* plus an adjective or a participle:

highly developed species   barely breathing bird
newly minted coins   easily seen result

3.23 Compounds with *better, best, ill, lesser, little, well,* and related comparative forms should be hyphenated when they precede the noun:

better-paid job   little-expected aid
best-liked teacher   well-intentioned man
ill-advised step   lesser-known evil

but

a very well intentioned man

As predicate adjectives, they are generally spelled as two words:

The step was ill advised.

It was clear that the man was well intentioned.

3.24 An adjective form composed of a present participle preceded by its object, or a past participle preceded by a related word, should be hyphenated:

emotion-producing language
thought-provoking commentary
dissension-arousing speeches
vote-getting tactics
foreign-made products
computer-formatted copy

Noun forms similarly constructed are generally treated as two words:

decision making   problem solving
coal mining   food gathering

3.25 Chemical terms used as adjectives are spelled as two or more words, unhyphenated:

44

```
boric acid solution          hydrogen sulfide gas
sodium chloride crystals     tartaric acid powder
```

3.26 Compounds with *all* should be hyphenated whether they precede or follow the noun:

```
all-encompassing aim     all-round leader
all-powerful ruler       all-inclusive title
all-pervasive evil       it was all-important
```

3.27 Hyphenate phrases used as adjectives before a noun:

```
six-to-ten-year-old group   matter-of-fact approach
on-the-job training         wage-price controls
catch-as-catch-can effort   fringe-benefit demands
```

3.28 Most adjectival compounds made up of an adjective plus a noun to which the suffix *ed* has been added should be hyphenated before the noun they modify and spelled as two words after the noun:

```
rosy-cheeked boy      fine-grained powder
straight-sided dish   open-handed person
```

but

```
A spot of pink made the boy appear rosy cheeked.

The president of the firm was known to be
extremely liberal minded.
```

3.29 Adjective forms ending with the suffix *like* should be spelled as one word except when they are formed from proper names, word combinations, or words ending with *l* or *ll:*

```
camplike       mouselike
museumlike     umbrellalike
```

but

```
barrel-like        doll-like
Cinderella-like    kitchen-cabinet-like
```

3.30 An adjectival compound composed of a cardinal number and the word *odd* should be hyphenated before or after the noun:

```
forty-odd    twenty-five-hundred-odd
175-odd      fifteen-hundred-odd
```

3.31 An adjectival compound composed of a cardinal number and a unit of measurement is hyphenated when it precedes a noun:

45

```
twelve-mile limit      eight-space indention
two-inch margin        hundred-yard dash
```

but

```
10 percent increase
```

3.32   Adjectival compounds with *fold* are written as one word unless numerals are used:

```
tenfold     multifold
```

but

```
20-fold
```

3.33   Noun compounds with *quasi* should be spelled as two words:

```
quasi promise     quasi honor
```

Adjectival compounds with *quasi* are hyphenated whether they come before or after the noun:

```
quasi-religious     quasi-political
```

3.34   Nowhere is the trend away from the use of hyphens more evident than in words with such common prefixes as *pre, post; anti; over, under; intra, extra; infra, ultra; sub, super; re; un; non; mini, maxi; micro, macro; multi; semi; pseudo; supra:*

```
prenuptial            subatomic
postoperative         supersonic
antirevolutionary     reenact
oversupplied          unconcerned
understaffed          macroeconomics
intramural            nonfunctional
extramural            semiconscious
infrared              pseudoreligious
ultraviolet           supramundane
```

Adjectives with these prefixes are spelled as one word unless the second element is capitalized or is a numeral:

```
pro-Arab     un-American     pre-1900
```

Or unless the form might be misleading or puzzling:

```
pro-choice     anti-utopian
```

Or unless the second element consists of more than one word:

```
non-food-producing people
pre-nuclear-age civilization
```

It is also necessary to distinguish homographs:

```
re-cover     recover
```

Division of Words

GENERAL RULES

3.35 Divide words at the ends of lines according to the syllabication shown in a reliable dictionary (preferably *Webster's Third New International Dictionary* or *Merriam-Webster's Collegiate Dictionary,* as suggested in 3.1).

3.36 Avoid ending more than two consecutive lines with hyphens.

3.37 Word processing programs that produce justified lines hyphenate automatically, sometimes responding to cues set in the copy to indicate preferred breaking points. Do not assume that automatic hyphenation programs always produce correct results. Most are not context sensitive and therefore cannot distinguish between *rec-ord* and *re-cord,* for example. Large spaces between words in formatted copy that has been justified by a computer must be closed up in the process of adjusting the hyphenation. Since an uneven, or ragged, right margin is acceptable for most research papers, it is best to avoid justification programs, which require special proofreading and checking of automatic hyphenation. If a paper is to be submitted for publication, the publisher will no doubt prefer unjustified copy for editing and typesetting.

3.38 Divide according to pronunciation rather than derivation. This means that when a word is divided after an accented syllable, the consonant stays with the vowel when the vowel is short:

```
signif-icant    param-eter    hypoth-esis
philos-ophy     democ-racy    pres-ent (noun)
```

But the consonant goes with the following syllable when the preceding vowel is long:

```
stu-dent    Mongo-lian    divi-sive
```

The consonant goes with the accented syllable, however, in such cases as the following:

```
philo-sophical    pre-sent (verb)    demo-cratic
```

3.39   Never divide a combination of letters pronounced as one syllable:

    pro-nounced   ex-traor-di-nary   passed

3.40   When *ing* or *ed* is added to a word whose final syllable contains the liquid *l* (e.g., *cir · cle, han · dle*), the final syllable of the parent word becomes a part of the added syllable:

    cir-cling   bris-tling   chuck-ling   han-dling
    cir-cled   bris-tled   chuck-led   han-dled

3.41   In words where a final consonant is doubled before *ing* and *ed,* the division comes between the double consonants:

    set-ting   con-trol-ling
    per-mit-ting   per-mit-ted

Note that this rule does not apply to words originally ending in a double consonant:

    add-ing   in-stall-ing

SPECIAL RULES

3.42   Some divisions, although syllabically correct, should never be made.

3.43   Never make a one-letter division:

Wrong:

    a-mong   u-nite   e-nough   man-y

3.44   Never divide the syllables *able* and *ible:*

Wrong:

    inevita-ble   permissi-ble   allowa-ble

Right:

    inevi-table   permis-sible   allow-able

3.45   Never divide the following suffixes:

    ceons   ceous   cial   cion
    geons   geous   gial   gion   gious
                      sial   sion
                      tial   tion   tious

48

3.46 Two-letter divisions are permissible at the end of a line, but two-letter word endings should not be carried over to the next line if this can be avoided:

```
en-chant     di-pole      as-phalt
```

but

```
losses (not loss-es)     stricken (not strick-en)
money (not mon-ey)       fully (not ful-ly)
```

3.47 Avoid dividing hyphenated words or compounds except at the hyphen:

Wrong:

```
self-evi-dent    gov-er-nor-elect    well-in-ten-tioned
```

3.48 Avoid dividing a proper name unless the correct division is obvious:

Right:

```
Wash-ing-ton    Went-worth    Bond-field    John-son
```

A source such as *Webster's New Biographical Dictionary* should be consulted before risking division of most proper names.

3.49 Never divide initials used in place of given names. It is best to write given names or initials on the same line as the family name, but it is allowable to place all the initials on one line and the family name on the next:

Wrong:

```
T. / S. Eliot     J. / B. S. Haldane
```

Allowable:

```
T. S. / Eliot     J. B. S. / Haldane
```

3.50 Never divide capital letters used as abbreviations for names of countries or states (U.S., N.Y.); for names of organizations (YMCA, NATO); or for names of publications or radio or television stations (*PMLA*, KKHI, KQED); but two sets of initials separated by a hyphen, such as KRON-FM, may be divided after the hyphen. Similarly, never divide the abbreviations for academic degrees (B.A., M.S., LL.D., Ph.D., etc.).

3.51 Never divide a day of the month from the month, and never divide any such combinations as the following:

```
£6 4s. 6d.      A.D. 1895      6:40 P.M.
245 ml          435 B.C.       10%
```

3.52 Never end a line with a divisional mark such as (*a*) or (1), a dollar sign, or an opening quotation mark, parenthesis, or bracket; and never begin a line with a closing quotation mark, parenthesis, or bracket.

3.53 For rules on word division in foreign languages, consult *The Chicago Manual of Style,* fourteenth edition, chapter 9.

PUNCTUATION

3.54 Punctuation in some of its specialized uses is treated elsewhere in this manual, in the chapters on abbreviations and numbers (2), quotations (5), tables (6), illustrations (7), notes (8), bibliographies (9), and parenthetical references and reference lists (10). Here the general use of the various marks of punctuation in the text is dealt with briefly, the primary aim being to answer questions that frequently puzzle writers. The rules are based on *The Chicago Manual of Style,* fourteenth edition. Note that in running text a single space follows any kind of terminal punctuation—periods, question marks, and exclamation points. (But see also under abbreviations, 2.2.)

Period

3.55 A period is used to end a declarative statement, a moderately imperative statement, or an indirect question, whether grammatically complete or only a sentence fragment.

Kathy sighed when she realized what had to be done.

Foolishness.

Carrie began to show signs of impatience.

Please, Carrie, be patient.

Hush.

Max winked at Ian and asked Carrie if something had upset her.

3.56 A period following an abbreviation and coming at the end of a sentence may serve also as the closing period of the sentence.

If the sentence ends with a question mark or an exclamation point, the abbreviation period is retained:

```
The meeting adjourned at 5:30 P.M.

Was the committee meeting called for 8:00 P.M.?
```

3.57   Periods are omitted at the ends of items in a vertical list or enumeration, unless the items are whole sentences or paragraphs.

```
The report covers three areas:
    1.  The securities markets
    2.  The securities industry
    3.  The securities industry in the economy
The course has three goals:
    1.  Emphasis is on the discovery of truth.
    2.  Emphasis is on the useful.
    3.  Emphasis is on love of people, especially the
        altruistic and philanthropic aspects of love.
```

3.58   Periods are omitted at the ends of all the following: (1) display headings for chapters, parts, and the like; (2) titles of tables; (3) captions of figures, unless the caption is run into a legend (see 7.14); (4) any subheading that is typed on a line by itself; and (5) address and datelines in communications, and also signatures.

3.59   A series of periods is used to mark omissions in quoted matter (ellipsis points; see chapter 5), and occasionally to guide the eye from items in one column of a table to relevant items in opposite columns (period leaders). Those who use computer formatting should be aware that certain programs that justify lines by altering the amount of space between characters or words on a line may require special steps to create ellipsis points and period leaders with uniform spaces between them. Such programs may also introduce two spaces after periods that are at the ends of lines in the unformatted copy, whether these periods end sentences or not.

QUESTION MARK

3.60   A question mark is used at the end of a whole sentence containing a query or at the end of a query making up part of a sentence:

```
Would the teacher-transplant idea catch on in countries
other than Germany? was the question the finalists
were asking.
```

```
The question put by the board was, Would the taxpayers
vote another bond issue that would raise taxes?
```

The first word of the sentence that asks the question is capitalized, even though it is included in another sentence, and quotation marks are generally unnecessary.

3.61 Courtesy disguises as questions such requests as the following, which should end with a period rather than a question mark:

```
Will you please submit my request to the appropriate
office.
```

3.62 A question mark may be used to indicate uncertainty:

```
The Italian painter Niccolò dell'Abbate (1512?-71)
assisted in the decorations at Fontainebleau.
```

EXCLAMATION POINT

3.63 An exclamation point marks an outcry or an emphatic or ironical comment (avoid overuse). Like the query (3.60), an exclamation may occur within a declarative sentence:

```
What havoc was wrought by hurricane Andrew!
```

```
"Incredible!" he exclaimed. "I could hardly believe my
senses. Both houses actually passed major bills on the
opening day!"
```

3.64 Do not use an exclamation point to call attention to an error in a quotation; place the word *sic* (italicized or underlined) in brackets after the error (see 2.25–26).

COMMA

3.65 Although the comma signals the smallest interruption in continuity of thought or sentence structure, when correctly used it contributes greatly to ease of reading and ready understanding.

3.66 In sentences containing two or more independent clauses joined by a coordinating conjunction (*and, but, or, nor, for*), a comma is placed before the conjunction. This is not a hard-and-fast rule, however; where the sentence is short and clarity is not an issue, no comma is needed.

```
Most young Europeans spend their holidays in other
European countries, and many students take vacation
jobs abroad.
```

```
This silence is not surprising, for in those circles
Marxism is still regarded with suspicion.
```

```
John arrived early and Mary came an hour later.
```

3.67 A comma is omitted before a conjunction joining the parts of a compound predicate (two or more verbs having the same subject):

```
The agencies should design their own monitoring
networks and evaluate the data derived from them.
```

```
They do not self-righteously condone such societies but
attempt to refute them theoretically.
```

3.68 In a series consisting of three or more elements, the elements are separated by commas. When a conjunction joins the last two elements, a comma is used before the conjunction.

```
Attending the conference were Farmer, Johnson, and
Kendrick.
```

```
We have a choice of copper, silver, or gold.
```

3.69 No commas should be used, however, when the elements in a series are all joined by the same conjunction:

```
For dessert the menu offered a choice of peaches or
strawberries or melon.
```

3.70 A series of three or more words, phrases, or clauses ending with the expression *and so forth* or *and so on* or *and the like* or *etc.* customarily has required commas both before and after the expression:

```
The management can improve wages, hours, conditions,
benefits, and so on, as part of the settlement package.
```

In its fourteenth edition, however, *The Chicago Manual of Style* accepts treating expressions like *etcetera* as the final item in the series and therefore not requiring a following comma.

```
Manfred regarded apologies, excuses, and the like as
barbarisms.
```

3.71   When commas occur within one or more of the elements of a series, semicolons should separate the elements:

> Three cities that have had notable success with the
> program are Hartford, Connecticut; Kalamazoo, Michigan;
> and Pasadena, California.

3.72   Commas are used to set a nonrestrictive dependent clause off from an independent clause. A clause is nonrestrictive if omitting it will not alter the meaning of the independent clause:

> These books, which are placed on reserve in the
> library, are required reading for the course.

Here omitting the dependent clause yields "These books are required reading for the course." But in the following sentence, the dependent clause identifies the books placed on reserve as "required reading for the course," and the clause is therefore restrictive. No commas should be used:

> The books that are required reading for the course are
> placed on reserve in the library.

3.73   A word, phrase, or clause in apposition to a noun may also be restrictive or nonrestrictive. When nonrestrictive, it is set off by commas:

> His brother, a Harvard graduate, transferred to
> Princeton for a program in theology.

> A onetime officer in the foreign legion, the man hoped
> to escape further military duty.

If, however, the appositive limits the meaning of the noun and is therefore restrictive, no commas should be used:

> The Danish philosopher Kierkegaard asked, "What is
> anxiety?"

> The motion picture *Becket* was adapted from the play by
> Jean Anouilh.

3.74   A title or position following a person's name should be set off with commas:

> Norman Cousins, former editor of the *Saturday Review*,
> wrote the editorial "Lunar Meditations."

3.75   The individual elements in addresses and names of places are set off with commas, except for zip codes:

> The address is 340 Forest Avenue, Palo Alto,
> California 94023.

```
The next leg of our trip was to take us to Springfield,
Illinois, and promised to be the most rewarding.
```

3.76 Interjections, conjunctive adverbs, and the like are set off with commas when they cause a distinct break in the flow of thought:

```
Nevertheless, it is a matter of great importance.

It is, perhaps, the best that could be expected.
```

But note that when such elements do not break the continuity and do not require a pause in reading, the commas should be omitted:

```
It is therefore clear that no deposits were made.
```

3.77 In using commas to set off a parenthetical element in the middle of a sentence, remember to include both commas:

```
The bill, you will be pleased to hear, passed at the
last session.
```

3.78 A comma follows *namely, that is, for example, i.e.,* and *e.g.* There must be a punctuation mark before each of these expressions, but the kind varies with the nature and complexity of the sentence:

```
Many people feel resentful because they think they have
suffered an unjust fate; that is, they look on illness,
bereavement, or disrupted domestic or working
conditions as being undeserved.

Restrictions on the sulfur content of fuel oil are
already in effect in some cities (e.g., Paris, Milan,
Rome, and Stockholm), and the prospect is that limits
will be imposed sooner or later in most cities.
```

3.79 When a dependent clause or a long participial or prepositional phrase begins a sentence, it is followed by a comma:

```
If the insurrection is to succeed, the army and the
police must stand side by side.

After spending a week in conferences, the commission
was able to write a report.

Having accomplished his mission, he returned to
headquarters.
```

But a comma is usually unnecessary after a short prepositional phrase:

```
For recreation the mayor fishes or sails.
```

3.80 When each of several adjectives preceding a noun modifies the
noun individually, the adjectives should be separated with
commas:

```
It was a large, well-placed, beautiful house.
```

```
We strolled out into the warm, luminous night.
```

However, if the last adjective *identifies* the noun rather than
merely modifying it, no commas should precede it:

```
His is the large brick house on the corner.
```

3.81 Use commas to set off contrasted elements and two or more
complementary or antithetical phrases or clauses referring to
a single word following:

```
The idea, not its expression, is significant.
```

```
The harder we run, the more we stay in the same place.
```

```
She delighted in, but was also disturbed by, her new
leisure and freedom.
```

```
It is a logical, if harsh, solution to the problem.
```

3.82 Use a comma to separate two identical or closely similar
words:

```
They marched in, in twos.
```

```
Whatever is, is good.
```

3.83 A comma is sometimes necessary to prevent misreading:

```
After eating, the lions yawned and then dozed.
```

SEMICOLON

3.84 A semicolon marks a greater break in the continuity of a sentence than does a comma. A semicolon should be used between the parts of a compound sentence (two or more independent clauses) when they are not connected by a conjunction:

```
More than one hundred planned communities are in
various stages of completion; many more are on the
drawing board.
```

3.85   If the clauses of a compound sentence are very long and have commas within them, they should be separated with semicolons even though they are connected by a conjunction:

> Although productivity per capita in United States industry is almost twice that in West European industry, Western Europe has an increasingly well educated young labor force; and the crucial point is that knowledge, which is transferable between peoples, has become by far the most important world economic resource.

3.86   When used transitionally between the clauses of compound sentences, the words *hence, however, indeed, then,* and *thus* should be preceded by a semicolon and followed by a comma:

> There are those who think of freedom in terms of social and economic egalitarianism; thus, reformist governments of the Left are inherently viewed with greater favor than the regimes of the Right.

Clauses introduced by the transitional adverbs *yet* and *so* are preceded by a comma:

> Elizabeth was out of the office when I called, so I left a message.

> There was some increase in intensity, yet the hypothesis was not confirmed.

3.87   For the use of the semicolon instead of a comma, see also 3.71.

Colon

3.88   The colon indicates a discontinuity of grammatical construction greater than that marked by the semicolon. Whereas the semicolon separates parts of a sentence that are of equal significance, the colon is used to introduce a clause or phrase that expands, clarifies, or exemplifies the meaning of what precedes it:

> Europe and America share similar problems: their labor forces cannot compete with those of Third World nations, and they depend on the Third World for critical raw materials.

> People expect three things of their governments: peace, prosperity, and respect for civil rights.

3.89   A colon should be placed at the end of a grammatical element introducing a formal statement, whether the statement is quoted or not. A colon is also used after *following* or *as follows* or *in sum* followed by illustrative material or a list:

```
The qualifications are as follows: a doctorate in
physics; five years' experience in a national
laboratory; and an ability to communicate technical
matter to a lay audience.
```

```
These immigrants all shared the same dream: they
thought they could create the City of God on earth in
their own lifetimes.
```

For the use of numbers to enumerate items in text, see 2.72.

3.90   As noted elsewhere in this manual, a colon is used between chapter and verse in scriptural references (2.46), between hours and minutes in notations of time (2.57), between the title and subtitle of a book or article (4.10 and 8.39), between place and publisher in footnotes and bibliographical references (8.55), and between volume and page numbers in citations (8.80, 8.99, 8.101, and 10.14).

DASH

3.91   The dash, which in printing is an elongated hyphen called an em dash, in typescript consists of two hyphens with no space between or on either side of them.

3.92   A dash or a pair of dashes enclosing a phrase may indicate a sudden break in thought that disrupts the sentence structure:

```
Rutherford--how could he have misinterpreted the
evidence?
```

```
Some of the characters in Tom Jones are "flat"--to use
the term E. M. Forster coined--because they
unfailingly act in accordance with a set of qualities
suggested by a literal interpretation of their names
(e.g., Squire Allworthy).
```

3.93   Interruptions or faltering speech may be indicated by dashes:

```
Later in chapter 25, Jane Eyre again answers only with
a gesture: "I reflected, and in truth it appeared to me
the only possible one: satisfied I was not, but to
please him I endeavored to appear so--relieved, I
```

```
certainly did feel; so I answered him with a contented
smile."
```

Faltering speech, especially in fictional dialogue, may also be indicated by three spaced ellipsis dots:

```
"Agatha," he said anxiously, "I never . . . no, no,
please believe me . . . but how can you think such a
thing!"
```

3.94 A dash may introduce an element that emphasizes or explains the main clause through repetition of one or more key words:

```
He asked where wisdom was to be found--"the wisdom
that is above rubies."
```

```
One is expected to cram all this stuff into one's
mind--cram it all in, whether it's likely to be useful
or not.
```

3.95 In a sentence that includes several elements referring to a word that is the subject of a final, summarizing clause, a dash may precede the final clause:

```
The statue of the man throwing the discus, the
charioteer at Delphi, the poetry of Pindar--all show
the culmination of the great ideal.
```

3.96 Use four hyphens to indicate missing letters (e.g., in citing from a text that is mutilated or illegible), leaving no space between the first and last hyphens and the existing part of the word:

```
We ha---- a copy in the library.
```

```
H----h? [Hirsch?]
```

In transcribing from incomplete texts in languages other than English, it may be customary to indicate the length of the break by using one hyphen for each missing or illegible character. In such cases, follow the practice set by scholars and editors within the discipline.

3.97 Use six hyphens to indicate a whole word omitted or to be supplied:

```
The vessel left the ------ of July.
```

PARENTHESES

3.98 The principal uses of parentheses in the text of a paper are (1) to set off parenthetical elements, (2) to enclose the source of a quotation or other matter when a footnote is not used for the purpose, and (3) to set off the numbers or letters in an enumeration (as in this sentence). The first use is a matter of choice, since both commas and dashes are also used to set off parenthetical material. In general, commas are used for material closely related to the main clause, dashes and parentheses for material more remotely connected:

```
The conference has (with some malice aforethought) been
divided into four major areas.
```

```
It is significant that in the Book of Revelation (a
book Whitehead did not like because of its bloody and
apocalyptic imagery), the vision of a new heavenly city
at the end of time has the divine light shine so that
the nations walk by it, and the "kings of the earth
shall bring their glory into it" (Rev. 21:22-26).
```

```
Each painting depicted some glorious, or vainglorious,
public occasion of the last hundred years; in each--a
formal diplomatic banquet, a victory parade, the
opening of the Burbank Airport in 1931 (clouded by a
phalanx of tiny Ford Trimotors)--the crowds of people
were replaced by swarms of ants.
```

BRACKETS

3.99 Brackets are used (1) to enclose any interpolation in a quotation (see 5.37) and (2) to enclose parenthetical matter within parentheses:

```
The book is available in translation (see J. R. Evans-
Bentz, The Tibetan Book of the Dead [Oxford: Oxford
University Press, 1927]).
```

3.100 Brackets may be used to enclose the phonetic transcription of a word:

```
He attributed the light to the phenomenon called
gegenschein ['gā-gən-ˌshīn].
```

OTHER PUNCTUATION MARKS

3.101 The use of quotation marks is described in paragraphs 5.11–17.

3.102 The hyphen, sometimes considered a mark of punctuation, is discussed in paragraphs 3.12–53 (compound words and word division) and paragraph 2.67 (inclusive numbers).

MULTIPLE PUNCTUATION

3.103 The term *multiple punctuation* means the conjunction of two marks of punctuation—for example, a period and a closing parenthesis. Where such conjunction occurs, certain rules must be observed concerning whether to omit one mark or the other (such as a period when an abbreviation ends a sentence; see 3.56) and which mark to put first when both are kept.

3.104 A comma is generally omitted following a stronger mark of punctuation:

If he had watched "What's My Line?" he would have known the answer.

She shouts "Where's the beef!" and we cut to a close-up of the hamburger.

3.105 Two marks of punctuation fall in the same place chiefly where quotation marks, parentheses, or brackets are involved.

3.106 In American usage, a final comma or period always precedes a closing quotation mark, whether it is part of the quoted matter or not. Question marks and exclamation points precede quotation marks if they are part of the quoted matter or follow if they pertain to the entire sentence of which the quotation is a part. Semicolons and colons follow quotation marks. (If the quoted passage ends with a semicolon or a colon in the original, the mark may be changed to a period or a comma to fit the structure of the main sentence.)

Every public official and every professional person is called on "to join in the effort to bring justice and hope to all our people."

Even this small advance begins to raise the question, "What in effect is our true image, our real likeness?"

Do we accept Jefferson's concept of "a natural aristocracy among men"?

Charged by a neighbor with criminal mistreatment of her child and threatened with police action, the woman retorted, "Just you call the police, and you'll regret it to your dying day!"

How dreadful it was to hear her reply--calmly--"We'll let the law decide that"!

He made the point that "in every human attitude and choice we make, we are taking an attitude toward

```
Everyman"; and then he enlarged on the point in a
particularly telling way.

Rome's planned subcenter, EUR, is "almost a self-
contained city": it governs itself and provides its
own services.
```

See also 5.17.

3.107   In fields, such as linguistics or philosophy, where it is the practice to use single quotation marks to set off special terms, a period or comma follows the closing quotation mark (see also 5.12):

```
Some contemporary theologians were proclaiming the
'death of God'.
```

In other uses of single quotation marks the period or comma is placed within the closing quotation mark (or marks, when both single and double occur together):

```
The article he referred to is in the Journal of
Political Economy: "Comment on 'How to Make a Burden of
the Public Debt.'"
```

3.108   When a complete sentence is enclosed in parentheses or brackets, the terminal period for that sentence is placed within them. When elements within a sentence are enclosed in parentheses or brackets, the sentence punctuation is placed outside.

```
We have already noted similar motifs in Japan.
(Significantly, very similar motifs can also be found
in the myths and folktales of Korea.)

Myths have been accepted as literally true, then as
allegorically true (by the Stoics), as confused history
(by Euhemerus), as priestly lies (by the philosophers
of the Enlightenment), and as imitative agricultural
ritual mistaken for propositions (in the days of
Frazer).
```

3.109   Numbers or letters in an enumeration run into the text belong with the items following them; therefore sentence punctuation precedes them, and no punctuation mark comes between them and the items they apply to:

```
He gave three reasons for resigning: (1) advanced age,
(2) failing health, and (3) a desire to travel.
```

3.110   Brackets used to set off words or phrases supplied to fill in incomplete parts of a quotation (5.35–37) or dates supplied in citations (8.68) are ignored in punctuating—that is, punctuate as if there were no brackets:

```
The states have continued to respond to "the federal
stimulus for improvement in the scope and amount of
categorical assistance programs. . . . [Yet] Congress
has adhered to its original decision that residence
requirements were necessary."
```

A WARNING FOR COMPUTER USERS

3.111 Punctuation marks may be part of the control language in a word processing program. To avoid costly errors, consult the documentation before entering any part of the paper. For example, some programs require control words that begin with periods, and these control words must often be introduced at the beginnings of lines. When using such programs, therefore, writers must avoid putting periods in the first character space in lines (e.g., for ellipses).

4 Capitalization, Italics, and Quotation Marks

Capitalization 4.1
  Proper Nouns 4.1
  Other Terms 4.4
  Titles of Works 4.5
    Headline-Style Capitalization 4.6
    Sentence-Style Capitalization 4.9
    Titles in Foreign Languages 4.10
    Parts of Works 4.13
Italics and Quotation Marks for Titles 4.14
  Books and Periodicals 4.16
  Series and Editions 4.18
  Dissertations and Other Unpublished Works 4.19
  Manuscript Collections 4.20
  Sacred Scriptures 4.21
  Legal Cases 4.22
  Poems 4.23
  Plays and Motion Pictures 4.24
  Radio and Television Programs 4.25
  Ships and Aircraft 4.26
  Other Nonbook Materials 4.27
Foreign Words and Phrases 4.28

CAPITALIZATION

PROPER NOUNS

4.1 In all languages written in the Latin alphabet, proper nouns—the names of persons and places—are capitalized:

    John and Jane Doe   Niagara Falls

4.2 In English, proper adjectives—adjectives derived from proper nouns—are also capitalized:

```
European     Machiavellian
```

4.3 Proper nouns and adjectives that have lost their original meanings and have become part of everyday language, however, are not capitalized:

```
french doors     india ink     roman numerals
```

OTHER TERMS

4.4 Before preparing the final manuscript, the writer should decide which terms are to be capitalized and which are not. Inconsistency in the matter may be a source of irritation and confusion. Detailed suggestions for capitalization of many terms are found in chapter 7 of *The Chicago Manual of Style,* fourteenth edition. The following paragraphs discuss capitalization of titles of written works, the problem encountered most frequently by writers of papers.

TITLES OF WORKS

4.5 In giving titles of published works in text, notes, reference list, or bibliography, the spelling of the original should be retained, but capitalization and punctuation may be altered to conform to the style used in the paper. In most scientific fields, sentence-style capitalization is used (see 4.9). In the humanities and many of the social sciences, however, it is customary to capitalize titles headline style, according to the rules given in 4.6–8.

HEADLINE-STYLE CAPITALIZATION

4.6 In the titles of works in English, capitalize the first and last words and all other words except articles, prepositions, *to* used as part of an infinitive, and coordinating conjunctions (*and, but, or, nor, for*):

Economic Effects of War on Women and Children

"What It Is All About"

How to Overcome Urban Blight: A Twentieth-Century Problem

Note that the subtitle, following a colon, is capitalized the same way as the main title.

4.7 Capitalizing compounds in titles may be simplified by the following rule: First elements are always capitalized; subsequent elements are capitalized unless they are articles, prepositions, or coordinating conjunctions.

Twentieth-Century Literature in the Making

Computer-Aided Graphics: A Manual for Video-Game Lovers

A Run-in with Authorities

There are a few cases that escape this perhaps oversimplified rule. For example, the modifiers *flat, sharp,* and *natural* following musical key symbols are not capitalized, and second elements attached to prefixes are capitalized only if they are proper nouns or proper adjectives.

Post-World War II Conflicts

E-flat Concerto

Strategies for Re-establishment

Mid-Atlantic Conference

The final element of a compound that comes at the end of a title (other than one with a hyphenated prefix), is always capitalized (see 4.6).

4.8 The original capitalization of titles of works published in earlier centuries may be retained:

A Treatise of morall philosophy Contaynyge the sayings of the wyse

SENTENCE-STYLE CAPITALIZATION

4.9 In reference lists, capitalize titles of books and articles sentence style; that is, capitalize the first word of the title or subtitle and only proper nouns and proper adjectives thereafter.

The triumph of Achilles

Seeing and selling America, 1945-55

"Natural crisis: Symbol and imagination in the American farm crisis"

TITLES IN FOREIGN LANGUAGES

4.10 In titles of foreign works, capitalize only what would be capitalized in a normal sentence. The first word of a subtitle is also capitalized. As with works in English, a colon should separate title and subtitle. If a period separates them, it should be changed to a colon:

Dictionnaire illustré de la mythologie et des antiquités grecques et romaines

Bibliografia di Roma nel Cinquecento

Historia de la Orden de San Gerónimo

Reallexikon zur deutschen Kunstgeschichte

Phénoménologie et religion: Structures de l'institution chrétienne

Since some romance language departments may have other rules for capitalizing titles, it is well to inquire before preparing the final manuscript.

4.11 In Latin and transliterated Greek titles, capitalize the first word and all proper nouns and proper adjectives thereafter:

Speculum Romanae magnificentiae

Iphigeneia hē en Taurois

4.12 An exception is made for modern works with Latin titles, which are capitalized as in English:

Acta Apostolicae Sedis   *Quo Vadis?*

PARTS OF WORKS

4.13 References in text to such parts of a work as contents, preface, foreword, introduction, bibliography, and appendix should not be capitalized:

A foreword may be included if desired.

The paper should include a bibliography.

The preface to this popular work was written by Lionel Trilling.

"Thinking French" is the title of chapter 6.

The variables within the experiment are listed in table 2.

Copies of supporting documents are in appendix 3.

ITALICS AND QUOTATION MARKS FOR TITLES

4.14 Throughout this manual, words that are italicized in examples may be underlined if italics are not available on the computer system or typewriter being used. Never use both italics and underlining in the same manuscript, however. The punctuation immediately following italics (except parentheses, brackets, or quotation marks) must also be italic.

4.15 In all fields except some of the sciences, titles of published books and some other kinds of works are italicized. Other titles are enclosed in double quotation marks, and still others are capitalized but neither italicized nor put in quotation marks. The general rule is to italicize the titles of *whole* published works and to put the titles of *parts* of these works in quotation marks. Titles of unpublished material are also put in quotation marks (see 4.16 and 8.130–32). Titles of series and manuscript collections, and various kinds of descriptive titles, are neither italicized not put in quotation marks (see 4.18–20).

BOOKS AND PERIODICALS

4.16 Italicize the titles of books, pamphlets, bulletins, periodicals (magazines, journals, newspapers), and long poems (such as *Paradise Lost*). Note that although published works are often thought of as being set in type and printed in conventional form, they may also include photocopied typescripts, works generated by desktop composition, or material in microform. *If the work bears a publisher's imprint,* it should be treated as published; that is, the title should be italicized wherever it appears (see also 8.130).

4.17 Titles of chapters or other divisions of a book and titles of short stories, short poems, essays, and articles in periodicals are put in quotation marks:

The First Circle, chapter 27, "A Puzzled Robot"

"The New Feminism," *Saturday Review*

"Amazing Amazon Region," *New York Times*

"The Demon Lover," in *Fifty Years: A Retrospective Collection*

Part 4 of *Systematic Theology,* "Life and the Spirit"

"The Dead," the final story in *Dubliners*

SERIES AND EDITIONS

4.18 Titles of series and names of editions are neither italicized nor put in quotation marks:

Michigan Business Studies

Modern Library Edition

DISSERTATIONS AND OTHER UNPUBLISHED WORKS

4.19 Titles of unpublished theses, dissertations, and other papers are put in quotation marks:

"Androgen Action and Receptor Specificity" (Ph.D. diss., University of Chicago, 1985)

"Costing of Human Resource Development," paper presented at the Conference of the International Economics Association

"One Man's CBI: A Different Kind of War," TMs, Hoover Library, Stanford, Calif.

MANUSCRIPT COLLECTIONS

4.20 Names of manuscript collections and archives, and designations such as *diary, autograph,* or *memorandum,* are not italicized or put in quotation marks when they occur in running text. In notes and bibliographical or reference list entries in papers citing many such primary sources, they should be put in roman and abbreviated, with the designations capitalized sentence style (see 2.19, 4.9, 8.131, 11.52–55).

SACRED SCRIPTURES

4.21 The titles of sacred scriptures—Bible, Qur'an (Koran), Talmud, Upanishads, Vedas, and the like—and the names of books of the Bible and of the Apocrypha are neither italicized nor put in quotation marks:

This passage is taken from the King James Version of the Bible.

The Book of Daniel is a part of the apocalyptic literature of the Bible.

LEGAL CASES

4.22 The names of legal cases (plaintiff and defendant) are italicized in text; *v.* (versus) may be in roman or italics, provided that use is consistent:

Miranda v. *Arizona*

Green v. *Department of Public Works*

West Coast Hotel Co. v. *Parrish*

POEMS

4.23 Titles of long poems are italicized; titles of short poems are put in quotation marks:

Milton's *Paradise Lost*

"Pied Beauty," in *The Oxford Book of Modern Verse*

Where many poems, both long and short, are mentioned, it is best to italicize all titles.

PLAYS AND MOTION PICTURES

4.24 Titles of plays and motion pictures are italicized:

Molière's *Le bourgeois gentilhomme*

Orson Welles's *Citizen Kane*

RADIO AND TELEVISION PROGRAMS

4.25 The title of a continuing series on radio or television is italicized, but the title of an individual episode in such a series is in roman, enclosed in quotation marks. Titles of made-for-television movies and of radio or television dramas of more than one episode are also italicized.

CBS's *Sixty Minutes*

National Public Radio's *All Things Considered*

"Riot in the Rec Room," last night's episode on *Quiet Suburbs, Unquiet Lives*

SHIPS AND AIRCRAFT

4.26 Names of ships, aircraft, and spacecraft are italicized. Designations of class or make are not:

SS *Constitution*	*Spirit of St. Louis*
HMS *Saranac*	*Apollo 13*

OTHER NONBOOK MATERIALS

4.27 For titles of other nonbook materials, see 8.130–47.

FOREIGN WORDS AND PHRASES

4.28 In running text in English, italicize foreign words and phrases that are not part of sentences or passages quoted in full:

Clearly, this leads to the idea of *Übermensch* and also to the theory of the *acte gratuit* and surrealism.

4.29 A quotation entirely in a foreign language is not italicized. In the following sentence, the words *le pragmatisme* within the English text should be italicized, but the words of the quotation, all in French, should not:

The confusion of *le pragmatisme* is traced to the supposed failure to distinguish "les propriétés de la valeur en général" from the incidental.

4.30 In the following foreign language quotation, the author of the quoted passage has italicized some words used as examples.

The person using the quotation in a paper written in English must observe the author's usage, since a quotation must always be reproduced exactly as it appears in the original:

> Reviewing Mr. Wright's book, Professor Nichols writes: "Quand j'ai dû analyser le style de Wright . . . j'ai été frappé par l'emploi ironique de ses prépositions et conjonctions causales (*à cause de, parce que,* etc.)."

4.31 Foreign titles preceding and sometimes following proper names, and foreign names of persons, places, institutions, and the like, are not italicized:

Père Grou	the Académie Française
the Puerto del Sol	the Gare du Nord
M. Jacquet, ministre des	the Teatro Real
travaux publics	the Casa de los Guzmanes
the Vienna Staatsoper	Place d'Italie

4.32 Foreign words that have become sufficiently anglicized to be listed in a good English dictionary should not be italicized:

> de facto   vis-à-vis   milieu   weltschmerz

4.33 The writer's appreciation of the needs of the audience the paper is intended for will govern whether to include the definition of a foreign word in text, in a note, or in an appendix. If a definition follows a foreign word or phrase within the text, the definition is put in parentheses or quotation marks:

> "I would like to eat," or *ena tuainu-iai,* "I wanted to eat."

> According to Sartrean ontology, man is always *de trop* (in excess).

In notes and appendixes, translations into foreign languages should follow 4.28 if they are several words or less in length, and 4.29–30 if they are longer.

5   Quotations

Permissions 5.1
   Plagiarism 5.2
   Accuracy 5.3
Prose 5.4
Poetry 5.6
Epigraphs 5.9
Quotations in Notes 5.10
Quotation Marks 5.11
Punctuation with Quotation Marks 5.17
Ellipses 5.18
   Omission within a Sentence 5.19
   Omission Following a Sentence 5.22
   Full Line of Ellipsis Points 5.24
   Capitalization of First Word 5.26
   When Not to Use Ellipsis Points 5.27
   Omissions in Foreign Language Quotations 5.29
Block Quotations 5.30
Interpolations 5.35
Italics for Emphasis 5.38

PERMISSIONS

5.1　The use of quotations within a research paper is a way of representing the continuity of research within a field and introducing the ideas of others by referring directly to their works. Quotations involving more than a few contiguous paragraphs or stanzas, and the use of anything in its entirety—a poem, an essay, a letter, a section of a book, an illustration, or sometimes a table—may exceed the limits of "fair use" as defined by the Copyright Act of 1976. Publishers, libraries, and others who

73

hold the rights to literary works do not interpret fair use uniformly. For example, some publishers and others holding copyright define fair use in terms of length, although the Copyright Act and the courts have defined it more generally, in terms of proper use to illustrate or support a point, of accurate transcription, and of proper credit given in notes or parenthetical references. Some publishers require permissions for lengthy quotations used in dissertations and some do not. Some librarians consider dissertations a form of publication and some do not. Bear in mind, however, that it is the courts, not the publishers, who are the authorities on fair use. For a thorough discussion of the subject, see chapter 4 in *The Chicago Manual of Style,* fourteenth edition.

PLAGIARISM

5.2 By definition, a research paper involves the assimilation of prior scholarship and entails the responsibility to give proper acknowledgment whenever one is indebted to another for either words or ideas. This chapter demonstrates how to include the words and ideas of others in a paper by quoting works accurately and attributing quotations and ideas to their authors in notes (chapter 8), bibliographies (chapter 9), and parenthetical references and reference lists (chapter 10). Failure to give credit is plagiarism. *The MLA Style Manual* offers a very useful perspective on the subject (see pp. 4–5 and 164).

ACCURACY

5.3 In general, direct quotations should correspond exactly with the original in wording, spelling, capitalization, and punctuation. Exceptions to the general rule are discussed below.

PROSE

5.4 Short, direct prose quotations should be incorporated into the text of the paper and enclosed in double quotation marks: "One small step for man, one giant leap for mankind." But in general a prose quotation of two or more sentences that runs to eight or more lines of text in a paper should be set off from the text in single-spacing and indented in its entirety four spaces from the left margin, with no quotation marks at the beginning or end. A quotation so treated is called a *block quotation*. Exceptions to this rule are allowable when, for emphasis or comparison, it is desirable to set off shorter quotations. Paragraph indention in the original text should be indicated by a four-space indention within a block quotation, but single-space between the paragraphs. When including material from different sources in a single block quotation, however, double-space between separate passages. (See also 5.30–34.)

5.5   Some word processing programs use control words for inserting block quotations and assigning note numbers to them. Before preparing the final manuscript, those using computers should read the instructions.

POETRY

5.6   Quotations of two or more lines of poetry are normally set off from the text, line for line as in the original, aligned on the left and centered on the page without quotation marks. They may be double- or single-spaced, following the alignment of the source as closely as possible:

```
              We are not the same you and
    i, since here's a little he
    or is
    it It
    ? (or was something we saw in the mirror)?

                    e. e. cummings,
                 "here's a little mouse) and"
```

5.7   If the lines of the poem are too long to be centered on the page, all the lines should be indented four spaces from the left margin, with runover lines indented another four spaces:

```
    A child said What is the grass? fetching it to me
        with full hands;
    How could I answer the child? I do not know what
        it is any more than he.

    I guess it must be the flag of my disposition, out
        of hopeful green stuff woven.

                 Walt Whitman, "Song of Myself"
```

5.8   It is sometimes desirable to insert a line or two of verse into
running text, as when making a critical examination of a poem.
Quotation marks are placed at the beginning and end of the
line or lines quoted, and if there is more than one line, a slash,
or virgule (/), with a space before and a space after, separates
them. When using the line justification function of a word processing program, it may be necessary to enter these spaces on
the formatted version or use special program abilities.

> In the valley the mariners find life's purposes reduced
> to the simple naturalistic proposition, "All things
> have rest, and ripen toward the grave; / In silence,
> ripen, fall, and cease."

EPIGRAPHS

5.9   When used at the heads of chapters, epigraphs are not enclosed
in quotation marks. The name of the author of the quotation
and the title of its source are given below the epigraph, flush
right:

> A storm of mosquitoes may create a noise like thunder.
>
> Old Chinese saying

> Heavy matters! Heavy matters! But look thee here, boy.
> Now bless thyself: thou met'st with things dying, I
> with things new-born.
>
> Shakespeare, *The Winter's Tale*

QUOTATIONS IN NOTES

5.10   Prose quotations of whatever length appearing within notes
are enclosed in quotation marks and run in:

> [1]"He leaves a terrible blank behind him and I have
> a horrid lonely feeling knowing that he is gone"
> (Field-Marshal Lord Alanbrooke, Diary, 18 April 1940
> [AMs, Personal Files]). Writing of Dill somewhat
> later, Brooke expressed a strong feeling of admiration
> and affection: "I know of no other soldier in the whole
> of my career who inspired me with greater admiration
> and respect. An exceptionally clear, well-balanced
> brain, an infinite capacity for work, unbounded charm

```
of personality, but, above all, an unflinching
straightness of character. . . . I owe him an infinite
debt for all I learned from him" (idem, "Notes on My
Life" [AMs, Personal Files], 2:66).
```

Verse quotations are set off or run in as in text.

QUOTATION MARKS

5.11 Direct quotations other than block quotations as described in paragraphs 5.30–34 require double quotation marks at beginning and end. If the quoted passage itself contains a quotation that is set off with double quotation marks, they must be changed to single quotation marks (see 5.16). In a block quotation, however, double quotation marks within the original matter are retained.

5.12 Double quotation marks are also used to set off titles (see 4.17 and 4.19) and single words, letters, or numbers in certain contexts:

```
Twenty-one papers were prepared under the topics
"Background," "Relation to Card Catalogs,"
"Techniques," "Standards," and "Applications."

The enumerations may be numbered "1," "2," "3," etc.
```

In some fields—linguistics, theology—it is accepted practice to use single quotation marks to set off words and concepts (see also 3.107):

```
kami 'hair, beard'

The variables of quantification, 'something',
'nothing', . . .
```

5.13 If a whole letter is quoted, including address and signature lines, it should all be set off as an indented block quotation, retaining the spelling, punctuation, emphasis, and spacing of the original:

```
              To my Lord the Lord Deputy of Calais

        Pleaseth you to understand that I humbly beseech
    your noble person that it may please you to give me
    leave to set up certain bills and notices touching
    my craft of writing, so that if within this town of
```

```
Calais there be any who should desire to have the
aforesaid art taught to their children, together
with the French tongue, that the residence of the
said your humble servant is at St. Omer; and thus
doing, my lord, I shall pray God for your good
prosperity.
                    J. Filleul (St. Clare Byrne 1981, 5:738)
```

5.14 In quoting an outline, set it off as an indented block quotation, retaining the spelling, punctuation, emphasis, and spacing of the original:

```
    Their outline for the third-year course is as
follows:

    III.  Predicate-element concept

        A.  Verb

            1.  Forms and uses of verb 'to be'

            2.  Tense

                a)  Present perfect

                b)  Past perfect⁴
```

In quoting an enumeration, do likewise:

```
    1.  Book selection

    2.  Arrangement and organization of the collection

    3.  Guidance to readers⁶
```

Introduce all such material in such a way as to make it clear that it *is* quoted and not the writer's own work. Lengthy material of this nature may belong in an appendix.

5.15 To quote material that includes headings and subheadings, use a block quotation and retain the spacing, indention, spelling, and punctuation of the original, being careful to cite the source in a note or a parenthetical reference:

```
                        CHAPTER II

          THE DEVELOPMENT OF A RACE RELATIONS
                   ACTION-STRUCTURE

          Race Relations in the British Isles:
               1700 to the First World War

    From the defeat of the Spanish Armada in 1588
until the abolition of slavery throughout the
British Empire in 1833, the economy of Britain was
```

```
tied, in some measure, to the fortunes of the
African slave trade. . . .
     Conservatives and liberals felt that this
dependency had always been a mistake.⁸
```

5.16 For a quotation within a quotation, single quotation marks are used; for another quotation within that one, double marks are again used; for yet another, single marks; and so on:

```
The chairman reported as follows:

     The mayor's representative has replied: "I am
     authorized by the Chamber of Commerce to make this
     offer, their provision stating, 'The jobs shall be
     made available provided that the committee
     guarantee all the means for receiving
     applications.' That guarantee has been made and a
     procedure outlined for taking job applications."
     Our thanks go to the mayor for his handling of our
     committee's request. (Guthrie Center 1987, 4)
```

PUNCTUATION WITH QUOTATION MARKS

5.17 Periods and commas should be placed inside quotation marks (even when the quotation marks enclose only one letter or figure); semicolons and colons go outside. Question marks and exclamation points should be placed outside quotation marks unless the question or exclamation is part of the quotation. In the first example below, the question is posed not within the quotation, but within the sentence as a whole, and the question mark belongs after the closing quotation mark. In the next two examples the question mark and the exclamation point clearly belong within the quotation marks. The rules apply equally to quotations within quotations (5.16), whether or not the quotations end at the same place.

```
How does he show "evil leading somehow to good"?

One may well ask, "Is it really necessary to lose the
world in order to find oneself?"

The cries of "Long live the king!" echoed down the
broad avenues.

"You speak, my friend, with a strange earnestness,"
said old Roger Chillingworth.

In Keats's "Ode on a Grecian Urn," the urn says,
"Beauty is truth, truth beauty."

Eva replied, "Did he really say, 'Nothing will come of
nothing'?"
```

> "I'm not convinced," said Tony, "that he really *meant* 'nothing.' "

> "Later," said Iris, "that 'nothing,' albeit frightening, was made light of."

> Rosa remarked, "Tom's 'What's nothing?' provoked outrage."

See also 3.103–10.

ELLIPSES

5.18 Any omission of words, phrases, or paragraphs in quoted matter is shown by ellipsis points, which are period dots, not asterisks (stars). There should be a space before each dot, unless the first dot is the period of an abbreviation or sentence, and a space after the last if a word follows. Since ellipsis points stand for words omitted from the quotation itself, they are always placed *within* quotation marks. When quotation marks either precede or follow ellipsis points, do not leave a space between the quotation mark and the dot (but see 5.27–28). With word processing programs that justify lines by adjusting spaces between words, ellipsis points may require special processing. For example, some programs when formatting automatically add two spaces after periods that occur at the end of lines in the unformatted text, whether or not they end sentences.

OMISSION WITHIN A SENTENCE

5.19 An omission within a sentence is shown by three spaced dots:

> In conclusion he stated, "What we require . . . is a new method."

5.20 If other punctuation comes immediately before the ellipsis, it is placed next to the word:

> "We are fighting for the holy cause of Slavdom; . . . for freedom; . . . for the Orthodox cross."

5.21 If other punctuation occurs immediately before a word that is preceded by ellipsis points, that punctuation mark is placed before the word, with the usual intervening space:

> "All this is not exactly in S's tradition . . . ; and it was not, as I recall, your style."

OMISSION FOLLOWING A SENTENCE

5.22 An omission following a sentence is indicated by four dots. The first, placed immediately after the last word, is the period:

> "When a nation is clearly in the wrong, it ought to say so. . . . I am only enunciating principles that we apply in our own case."

If in the original source the sentence preceding the ellipsis ends with a question mark or an exclamation point, that mark rather than the period is used:

> "How cold it was! . . . No one could function in that climate."

5.23 How much of an omission may be indicated by a mark of terminal punctuation and three dots? In current practice, the period (or other mark of terminal punctuation) and three spaced dots may indicate the omission of (1) the last part of a quoted sentence, (2) the first part of a quoted sentence, (3) the last part of one sentence and the first part of the next sentence, (4) a whole sentence or more, or (5) a whole paragraph or more. But note the following exceptions.

FULL LINE OF ELLIPSIS POINTS

5.24 In quoting an excerpt of poetry, the omission of one or more complete lines is shown by a full line of ellipsis points, approximating in length the line of poetry immediately above it:

> Weep no more, woeful shepherds, weep no more,
> For Lycidas your sorrow is not dead,
>
> . . . .
> Henceforth thou art the genius of the shore,
> In thy large recompense, and shalt be good
> To all that wander in that perilous flood.[7]

5.25 The use of a full line of ellipsis points may be desirable in quoting portions of an outline or an enumeration. In the following example, the four dots at the end of the first paragraph indicate the omission both of the last part of item 1 and of items 2 and 3. The full line of dots that follows is necessary to indicate missing lines. The semicolon and the three dots at the end of item 4 indicate the omission of the last part of the paragraph.

```
1.  The paper must include a discussion of the moral
    bases and social effects of the kind of ownership
    which you favor or which you wish to attack. . . .

      .  .  .  .  .  .  .  .  .  .  .  .  .  .  .  .  .

4.  In form, the paper must be an argument: . . . . .
```

See also 5.23 and 5.34.

CAPITALIZATION OF FIRST WORD

5.26 Exact quotations should follow precisely the wording, spelling, capitalization, and punctuation of the original (5.3), but long-established scholarly practice makes an exception by altering the capitalization of the first word of a quotation according to the following rule:

1. If the quotation is set off syntactically from the text by a comma, period, or colon, the first word is capitalized, even though it is lowercase in the original.

```
The following day Sand reported, "With Pebble
soliciting members on the side, it was imperative that
the meeting be delayed no longer."
```

In the original of the passage above, "With" occurs within a sentence and is therefore not capitalized.

2. If, however, the quotation is joined syntactically to the writer's introductory words, the first word of the quotation is begun with a small letter, even if it is capitalized in the original:

```
The act provided that "the general counsel of the board
shall exercise complete supervision."
```

In the original, "the" is the first word of the sentence and is therefore capitalized. It is necessary to bracket such changes only in legal works and textual criticism.

WHEN NOT TO USE ELLIPSIS POINTS

5.27 In general, no ellipsis points should be used (1) before or after an obviously incomplete sentence, (2) before or after a run-in quotation of one or more complete sentences, (3) before a block quotation, or (4) after a block quotation ending with a complete sentence. If ellipsis points are considered necessary before or after a quoted passage, three should precede and four, including the period, follow the quoted matter if it ends with a complete sentence or if it ends the sentence in the text.

5.28 When a quotation consists of a few words or an incomplete sentence, obviously a fragment from the original, no ellipsis points should be used either before or after it. If, however, an omission occurs within the fragment, it is noted by three ellipsis points:

```
General Smith wrote that the president had been "very
much impressed" by the State Department's paper that
stressed "developing a major part of the world by using
the economic resources . . . of the superpowers."¹³
```

OMISSIONS IN FOREIGN LANGUAGE QUOTATIONS

5.29 Treat omissions in foreign language quotations as you would those in English. If the paper itself is written in a language other than English, follow the rules of that language in the matter of omissions (as well as for punctuation). Some of these rules are given in *The Chicago Manual of Style,* fourteenth edition.

BLOCK QUOTATIONS

5.30 When material in a block quotation (5.4) begins with a paragraph in the original, it is given a paragraph indention of four spaces and the first word is capitalized. Thus with a block quotation indented four spaces from the left margin, the paragraph indention is eight spaces from the left margin. (See also 5.32.)

```
Goodenough raises questions that Kraeling does not
raise:
        Primarily why did the artist want to put David
    as the tamer just here? We have seen that the
    original vine or tree growing from the vase was
    changed to highlight its naturalistic aspects, to
    make it more central to the composition, and to
    emphasize its derivation, thus making more explicit
    the symbolic and ritualistic implications of the
    vase. (Goodenough 1986, 40)
```

Note that the source directly follows the terminal punctuation of the quotation.

5.31   If a block quotation is introduced in text with quoted fragments interspersed with the words of the writer of the paper,
the fragments cited must all have quotation marks at beginning
and end. It is not permissible to begin a quotation within the
text with quotation marks, as required, and to continue the
quotation in block form, omitting quotation marks. Note
the following example of *incorrect usage* in introducing a
block quotation:

```
Religion is just "the product of the craving to know

whether these imaginary conceptions have realities

answering to them in some other world than ours." And

Mill continues: "Belief in a God or Gods

     and in a life after death becomes the canvas which
     every mind . . . covers with such ideal pictures as
     it can either invent or copy.⁶
```

Avoid introducing in running text a quotation that would have
to be completed in block form. The following illustrates *correct* usage:

```
And Mill continues:

     Belief in a God or Gods and in a life after death
     becomes the canvas which every mind . . . covers
     with such ideal pictures as it can either invent
     or copy.⁶
```

Sometimes the writer must rephrase the text or reconsider how
much to quote.

5.32   Two conditions under which a block quotation begins with
paragraph indention are considered in 5.30 and 5.33. Otherwise the first line of the block quotation is indented four spaces
from the left margin, as shown in the last example in 5.31. Note
that the first (partial) paragraph is the only one in a block quotation of more than one paragraph that may start flush left.
All the others must be given paragraph indention, whether the
quotation begins with the first sentence of the paragraph or at
some point within it.

5.33   If in a quotation of several paragraphs a full paragraph or
more is omitted, that omission should be indicated by a period
and three ellipsis points at the end of the preceding paragraph.
Thus four dots at the end of a paragraph may be followed by

three dots at the beginning of the next paragraph, as illustrated in the following example. Two consecutive sets of ellipsis points may occur in a block quotation, but not in a quotation that is run into text:

```
Recalling as an adult the time in his early youth when

a "new conscience" was forming, Merton writes:

        A brand-new conscience was just coming into
    existence as an actual, operating function of a
    soul. My choices were just about to become
    responsible. . . .
        . . . since no man ever can, or could, live by
    himself and for himself alone, the destinies of
    thousands of other people were bound to be
    affected, some remotely, but some very directly and
    near-at-hand, by my own choices and decisions and
    desires, as my own life would also be formed and
    modified according to theirs.⁷
```

5.34   If it is considered desirable to quote in block form fragments of prose that are widely scattered in the original source, a full line of ellipsis points may be used between the individual fragments.

INTERPOLATIONS

5.35   It is sometimes advisable to insert in a quotation a word or more of explanation, clarification, or correction. All such insertions, or interpolations, must be enclosed in brackets [ ]. Parentheses may *not* be substituted. Seeing a parenthetical element in a quotation, a reader assumes it was put there by the author of the source quoted. Brackets indicate that the comment was added by the person quoting the author. If the keyboard has no brackets, leave space and insert them in the copy by hand, in black ink.

5.36   To assure the reader that any faulty logic, error in fact, wrong word, incorrect spelling, or the like is in the original, the Latin word *sic* ("so," always in italic, without a period) may be placed in brackets after the error:

```
Little lizards gambling [sic] in the sun.
```

Sic should not be overused. Quotations from obviously archaic or nonstandard writing should not be strewn with *sic*s.

5.37   Interpolations made for clarification or correction are illustrated in the following:

> "But since these masters [Picasso, Braque, Matisse]
> appeared to be . . . rebelling against academic
> training, art teaching has itself been discredited."[4]

> "The recipient of the Nobel Peace Award for 1961 [1960]
> was Albert John Luthuli."[5]

ITALICS FOR EMPHASIS

5.38 Words that are not italicized in the original may be italicized (or underlined) for emphasis by the writer of the paper. The source of the change should be shown in one of three ways.

1. By a notation in brackets placed immediately after the italicized words:

> "This man described to me another large river beyond
> the Rocky Mountains, *the southern branch* [emphasis
> mine] of which he directed me to take."[7]

2. By a parenthetical note following the quotation:

> "This man described to me another large river beyond
> the Rocky Mountains, *the southern branch* of which he
> directed me to take" (emphasis mine).[7]

3. By a note. Either a note or the method in (2) is preferable when italics have been added at two or more points in a quotation.

6   Tables

Planning and Constructing Statistical Tables 6.3
Arrangement of the Elements 6.12
   Numbering 6.13
   Position 6.18
   Size and Shape 6.20
      Long and Narrow 6.21
      Wide 6.22
      Continued Tables 6.25
   Title 6.26
   Column Headings 6.33
   Stub 6.39
   Omissions 6.43
   Alignment 6.46
Abbreviations and Symbols 6.48
Footnotes 6.50
Ruling 6.59

6.1   Tables efficiently organize and compress data into a standard-ized form. Because tables must be accurate and easy to read, care is required in spacing, ruling, arrangement of headings, and placement with respect to the text. Because they supple-ment the text, tables should be within the text or in an appen-dix, unless they occupy a separate section.

6.2   Computer software that includes functions for managing spreadsheets, column adjustments, and other tabulation for-mats can be useful for designing tables. Some programs can generate rules and insert special characters such as "corners" for joining horizontal and vertical lines, although tables de-signed using software without such features can be treated just like typewritten tables, with any vertical rules inserted by hand (see 7.27–32). For more information on the use of software to compose tables and insert them in text, see 13.19–20.

PLANNING AND CONSTRUCTING STATISTICAL TABLES

6.3   Most tables that present information in numerical form—percentages, tallies of occurrences, amounts of money, and the like—are known as statistical tables. As a simple example, say a scholar has completed a survey on smoking among American adults, incorporating information on the respondents' date of birth, sex, income, social background, and the like, and wishes to present some of the data in tabular form. The survey has produced responses from 7,308 individuals—3,362 males and 3,946 females—all eighteen or over.

6.4   In any one table, a single category of responses is always the center of attention. The table is constructed to illustrate the variations in that category (the dependent variable) with respect to some other set or sets of data (independent variables). Here the dependent variable would be whether the respondent smoked, and the independent variable could be any of several other categories or facts, say the person's sex. Classifying responses according to these two variables might then result in the simple array shown in table 1. (The survey, needless to say, is imaginary, and all the data shown are entirely hypothetical.)

Table 1. Smokers and Nonsmokers, by Sex

	Smoke	Don't Smoke	Total
Males	1,258	2,104	3,362
Females	1,194	2,752	3,946
Total	2,452	4,856	7,308

6.5   An array of raw data like this is relatively useless, however. For comparison the data must be presented in terms of percentages. This has been done in table 2. In any statistical table employing percentages (or other proportional figures) the compiler should always give the finite number—the *database,* or N—from which the percentages are derived. Here N is given in a separate column, but other arrangements are also appropriate (see table 6).

6.6   Table 2 represents an extremely simple statistical situation. Both the independent variable (sex) and the dependent variable (smoke/don't smoke) are *dichotomies*—entities that divide into two mutually exclusive categories. When either variable consists of more than two categories, tabular presentation becomes more complex.

Table 2. Smokers and Nonsmokers, by Sex

	N	Smoke	Don't Smoke
Males	3,362	37.4%	62.6%
Females	3,946	30.3%	69.7%
Total	7,308	33.6%	66.4%

6.7   Say the researcher wishes to present the data in terms of age rather than sex. For this purpose birth dates would be grouped by years or spans of years to represent respondents' ages at the time of the survey, and these groups would be divided according to the smoke/don't smoke dichotomy. The results could be presented as in table 3. Here age is broken down into four categories, the first three consisting of fifteen-year spans, but smaller groupings could be used.

Table 3. Smoking among American Adults, by Age

Age	N	Smoke (%)	Don't Smoke (%)
18-32	1,722	30.6	69.4
33-47	2,012	37.1	62.9
48-62	1,928	35.2	64.8
63+	1,646	30.5	69.5
Total	7,308		

6.8   If the writer wishes to present the data by both age and sex, the responses would be subdivided once more. The data might then be presented as in table 4.

Table 4. Smoking among American Adults, by Age and Sex

Age and Sex	*N*	Smoke (%)	Don't Smoke (%)
Males			
18–32	792	30.0	70.0
33–47	926	44.9	55.1
48–62	886	34.5	65.5
63+	758	39.3	60.7
Total (males)	3,362		
Females			
18–32	930	31.0	69.0
33–47	1,086	30.4	69.6
48–62	1,042	35.7	64.3
63+	888	23.0	77.0
Total (females)	3,946		
Total (both)	7,308		

6.9   Suppose respondents were asked other questions about smoking—whether they had quit smoking or had ever tried to quit and (if they smoked at all) whether they smoked cigarettes. Presenting these data in meaningful ways involves expanding the tabular display and making it more complicated.

6.10   Take the data on quitting smoking. If these statistics are to be presented in connection with age and sex as the independent variables, they might be arranged as in table 5. Here each half of the basic smoke/don't smoke dichotomy has been further split according to whether or not the respondent has quit smoking or has tried to quit. The *N* for each age group also must be split between smokers and nonsmokers. Note that each column of *N*s applies to the two columns to the right of it.

6.11   Finally, let us say the writer wants to present data on cigarette smoking in connection with an element of social background—whether the respondent came from a rural, small town, or big city environment—as well as age and sex. (The question eliciting this response would of course have to be a definite one, such as "Which of these categories comes closest to the type of place you were living in when you were sixteen years old?" followed by a listing of various kinds of locales.) Responses are sorted first by age and sex, as for table 4, then

Table 5. Smoking History of American Adults, by Age and Sex

	Smoke			Don't Smoke		
	N	Have Tried to Quit (%)	Never Tried to Quit (%)	N	Never Smoked Regularly (%)	Quit Successfully (%)
Males						
18-32	238	15.1	84.9	554	93.9	6.1
33-47	416	28.8	71.2	510	72.2	27.8
48-62	306	60.1	39.9	580	46.6	53.4
63+	298	88.6	11.4	460	38.7	61.3
Total (males)	1,258	48.0	52.0	2,104	63.5	36.5
Females						
18-32	288	18.8	81.2	642	40.3	59.7
33-47	330	28.5	71.5	756	68.5	31.5
48-62	372	62.4	37.6	670	50.4	49.6
63+	204	89.2	10.8	684	41.8	58.2
Total (females)	1,194	47.1	52.9	2,752	62.6	37.4
Total (both)	2,452	47.6	52.4	4,856	45.2	54.8

by background of the respondent, with "Don't know" answers omitted. The twenty-four groups created by dividing the responses this way constitute the database for the final dichotomy of those who smoke cigarettes and, by elimination, everybody else (table 6). As before, the total in each category is expressed as a percentage of N. Here it is impractical to show Ns in columns of their own, so another device has been adopted: the N for each category is shown in parentheses below and slightly to the right of the percentage. Other arrangements are possible, but this one is preferred by most people who work with statistics.

ARRANGEMENT OF THE ELEMENTS

6.12   The conventions governing the arrangement of the various elements of a statistical table, though not immutable, are accepted by many who make frequent use of tables. Consequently, it is wise to follow existing fashions in the basics of tabular presentation.

NUMBERING

6.13   Every table should be numbered with an arabic numeral and given a title, even though there may be few tables in the paper. (However, a very simple tabulation—five or six figures arranged in two columns—introduced in such a way that a heading seems unnecessary, need not be given a number or a title.) The order in which the tables are mentioned in the text determines the numbering, which continues straight through all chapters.

6.14   Tables in an appendix should be numbered separately from the tables in the text, as A1, A2, and so on.

6.15   All text references to a table should be by number, not by an introductory phrase such as "in the following table."

6.16   The reference may be in running text or in parentheses:

```
The percentages in table 5 illustrate this margin of
error.

A majority of voters were absent during the election
(see table 4).

In table 25, the rates increase markedly.
```

Table 6. Smoking among Adult Americans, by Type of Background,
Urban or Rural

	Country (%)	Town or Small City (%)	Big City and Suburbs (%)
Males			
18-32	26.5	29.6	29.9
	(98)	(294)	(398)
33-47	34.6	41.2	43.0
	(153)	(306)	(460)
48-62	28.6	31.4	34.1
	(220)	(385)	(270)
63+	34.8	35.1	36.5
	(273)	(279)	(189)
Total (males)	31.8	34.2	36.3
	(744)	(1,264)	(1,317)
Females			
18-32	28.4	31.0	31.5
	(116)	(348)	(463)
33-47	27.9	30.6	31.1
	(179)	(359)	(540)
48-62	27.7	35.8	42.3
	(260)	(450)	(319)
63+	21.5	23.1	25.8
	(329)	(325)	(213)
Total (females)	25.6	30.6	32.8
	(884)	(1,482)	(1,535)
Total (both)	28.4	32.2	34.4
	(1,628)	(2,746)	(2,852)

Note: Figures in parentheses are base *N*s for the adjacent percentages. Total *N* = 7,226 (3,325 males, 3,901 females). Respondents (82) who did not know where they were living at age 16 have been excluded from the database.

6.17   Numbered references make it possible to set the table at the end of the page or the paragraph, or on a separate page, as its size permits.

POSITION

6.18   Ideally, each table should come as close as possible after the first reference to it. If space permits, however, it is best to finish the paragraph of text in which the reference occurs before inserting the table (see sample 14.31). If a table cannot be accommodated in the space remaining on a given page, continue the text to make a full page and place the table at the top of the next page.

6.19   If a table appears on a text page, three blank lines should be left above it and three blank lines below (i.e., the table number is typed on the fourth line following the text, and the text is continued on the fourth line below the bottom rule or the table's notes, as in sample 14.31).

SIZE AND SHAPE

6.20   In most tables the columns run the long way on the page. A table may occupy the full width of the page or less than the full width. In either case, each table must be centered horizontally on the page.

LONG AND NARROW

6.21   When a table is long and narrow, space may be saved and appearance enhanced by doubling it up—dividing it into equal parts and placing them side by side, repeating the stub and the column heads (see sample 14.26). A vertical rule separates the two sides.

WIDE

6.22   If a table is too wide for the page, it should be turned lengthwise (*broadside table;* see sample 14.30)—the table is entered using software that creates broadsides, or the paper is put in the typewriter sideways and the table is typed so that the columns run the short way of the paper. No text should be placed on a page containing a broadside table. The page number appears in its usual place, whether the paper is prepared on a typewriter or on a computer system.

6.23 A table too wide to be accommodated broadside may be arranged vertically on two facing pages. This is done by turning the first page over so that the text is on the back and thus faces the next page (the front of the first page remains blank). If the paper is to be bound, a note to the binder will ensure correct placement. The parts of the table must have the same dimensions on both pages, and special care is needed to align the figures in each column exactly with the appropriate items in the stub. If software will not automatically generate a wide table on facing pages, it may be possible to construct two table sections that can be mounted on opposite pages and then photocopied. A better solution might be to print out the table in smaller type or to reduce a standard printout photographically. This reduction can then be mounted on the page and photocopied, with its page number typed in the upper right corner. The type must be large enough to be legible in the microfilm reproduction of a thesis or dissertation.

6.24 Tables too wide to be accommodated on the 8½-by-11-inch page in the ways described above may be typed on a larger sheet and then folded, though this method is less satisfactory for dissertations that must be bound (see 7.44–46).

CONTINUED TABLES

6.25 Long tables may be continued from page to page. The table number and the title are placed at the beginning of the table; the table number only is given on succeeding pages, written, for example, "Table 2—*Continued.*" Ordinarily the column headings are repeated on every page, except that in a continued broadside table in which the pages face each other, the headings need not be repeated on the second page (and the fourth,sixth, etc.). In a table that is continued, the bottom rule is omitted except on the last page, at the end of the table.

TITLE

6.26 Each numbered table must have a title. If a very brief tabulation is introduced in such a way that a title seems unnecessary, the tabulation should not be given a table number (see 6.13).

6.27 Place the table number above the table at the left margin; add a period and continue with the title, running the first line and succeeding full lines the width of the table, single-spaced, and centering the last, shortest line. The title may be capitalized either headline style (see 4.6–8) or sentence style (see 4.9):

```
Table 21. Probable rate of damage per foot-candle
   for thirty light sources expressed in percentage
               relative to zenith day
```

Use one style of capitalization consistently in table titles throughout the paper.

6.28 In a traditional alternative style, the word TABLE in full capitals and the number in arabic numerals are centered. A blank line follows, and the table title, in capitals, is then centered, with any subheading centered on the next line (often in parentheses), capitalized headline style. If a title is longer than the width of the table, type it in two or more lines, arranged in an inverted pyramid and single-spaced (see samples 14.25–26, 14.28, and 14.30). If table titles contain chemical, physical, or mathematical expressions conventionally expressed in lowercase, these expressions should remain lowercase even though the rest of the title is in capitals. Or follow the style recommended in 6.27; but use one style consistently throughout the paper.

6.29 The title should identify the table briefly. It should not furnish background information or describe the results illustrated. For example,

```
Effect of DMSO on Arthritic Rats and Nonarthritic Rats
after 20, 60, and 90 Days of Treatment
```

should be pared down to something like

```
Effect of DMSO on Rats
```

The column headings indicating 20, 60, and 90 days and the horizontal rows for arthritic and nonarthritic rats will give the variables. Also, the kind of editorial comment implied by a title like

```
High Degree of Recidivism among Reform School Parolees
```

should be eliminated.

```
Recidivism among Reform School Parolees
```

is sufficient. A table should merely give facts; discussion and commentary belong in the text.

6.30 The title should be substantival in grammatical form. Avoid relative clauses in favor of participles. Not

```
Number of Families That Subscribe to Weekly
News Magazines
```

but rather,

```
Families Subscribing to Weekly News Magazines
```

6.31 In conservative practice *percent* is still not considered a noun, although colloquially it is commonly so used. Accordingly, rather than

```
Percent of cases diagnosed correctly
```

use

```
Percentage of cases diagnosed correctly
```

6.32 The table title may carry a subheading, often in parentheses:

```
Table 36. Investment in Automobiles since 1900
              (in Thousands of Dollars)
```

The number of individuals in a group under consideration (for example, $N = 253$) may be treated as a subheading if it applies to the whole table.

Column Headings

6.33 A table must have at least two columns and usually has more. The columns carry *headings* or *heads* at the top, brief descriptions of the material they contain.

6.34 Like the table title, the column headings are substantival in form. If the first column of a table (the *stub,* discussed below) carries a heading, it should be singular. The other headings may be singular or plural according to sense.

6.35   Column heads may carry subheadings when they are needed, usually to indicate the unit of measure employed. Subheadings are normally enclosed in parentheses; abbreviations, if used consistently throughout a series of tables, are acceptable: ($), (lb.), (%), (mi.), (× 100 km), (millions), and so on. If the columns of a table must be numbered for text reference, arabic numerals are put in parentheses as subheads.

6.36   Tabular matter sometimes demands two or more levels of headings, and then *decked heads* must be used. A decked head consists of a *spanner head* and the two or more column heads it applies to. A horizontal rule is set between spanner and column heads to show what columns the spanner covers (see sample 14.27). Decked heads should seldom exceed two levels, since larger ones are hard to follow down the columns of an unruled table.

6.37   Excessive decking of the heads can sometimes be avoided by using a *cut-in head*—a heading that cuts across the statistical columns of the table and applies to all the tabular matter lying below it. For an example of cut-in heads, see sample 14.28.

6.38   In typing column heads, leave at least two spaces between the longest lines in adjacent headings. The width of the column headings generally determines the total width of a table, so they should be kept as brief as possible. Use either headline- or sentence-style capitalization, and type runover lines flush left. Spanner and cut-in heads, however, must be centered above the columns they pertain to. The column head with the most lines defines the vertical space available for all the heads. In typing, it is simplest to align the last lines of all the other heads horizontally with the last line of the longest one. Any subheads are typed on the line below this one. Rules running the full width of the table are customarily typed or drawn above and below the column heads and any spanners used. The rule below a spanner head is exactly as wide as the column headings spanned, and the rules above and below a cut-in head are exactly as wide as the column heads they apply to (usually just the statistical columns, but sometimes the first column, or stub, as well, as in sample 14.28).

STUB

6.39   The left-hand column of a table, known as the stub, generally has a column heading unless the table title makes its contents clear. Items in the stub should be capitalized sentence style, and no periods are used at the ends of items. If items require runover lines, the items are single-spaced and runovers are indented three spaces. When an item is subdivided, however, the subdivisions are indented three spaces and any runovers are indented five spaces.

```
Relative to issue
    price
    1923-27 . . . . . . . . . . . . . . .
    1949-55 . . . . . . . . . . . . . . .
```

Another way to show subdivision in a stub is to italicize or underline the main entry but not the subdivisions, aligning all at the left (sample 14.29).

6.40   Consistency within the stub is also important. Items that are logically similar should be similarly phrased: Authors, Publishers, Printers, *not* Authors, Publishing concerns, Operates printshop. In a series of tables, the same item should always bear the same name in the stub: the Union of Soviet Socialist Republics, for instance, should not appear as USSR in one table and Soviet Union in another.

6.41   If *Total, Mean,* or *Average* appears in the stub, the word should be indented two spaces more than the greatest indention above it. If both *Total* and *Grand total* are given, the latter is indented farther.

6.42   If the open space between the end of a line in the stub and the columnar matter it refers to is such that the eye does not move easily from one to the other, period leaders (spaced periods) may connect the two (see 3.59).

OMISSIONS

6.43   If all figures in a column begin with a zero to the left of the decimal point, all the zeros may be omitted. Unless they are part of the column heading, degree and dollar signs must appear in the first entry in each column where they apply and after every break in a column, such as rules above totals and cut-in headings.

6.44 If all the figures in a table are in thousands or millions, space may be saved by omitting the zeros and noting the units in a subtitle; for example, "(Figures in Millions)." (See sample 14.29.)

6.45 A blank cell in a column should be indicated by at least three spaced period leaders, centered with respect to the longest number in the column (see sample 14.27), or the number necessary to occupy the full width of the column. Two hyphens may also be used. Follow one of these styles consistently.

ALIGNMENT

6.46 The items in the stub must be aligned with their related items in the columns. If the stub item occupies more than one line and the column entry only one, align on the last line of the stub (see sample 14.27); if both contain more than one line, align on the first line and omit leaders:

```
Mean water content
  (percent) . . . . . . . . . . . . . . . . 69.6
```

but

```
C₂ (35"-50"+) (fresh till,      Dark grayish brown (10 YR
    slightly oxidized)              4/2) bouldery loamy
                                   sand; massive structure;
                                   pH of 6.42
```

6.47 Align a column of figures vertically on the decimal points or commas (figures of 1,000 or more should have commas; see 2.66). Dollar signs and percent signs are aligned (see also 6.43). Mathematical operational signs $(+, -, <, =,$ etc.) are aligned if they precede quantities.

ABBREVIATIONS AND SYMBOLS

6.48 Although discouraged for the most part in text, abbreviations and symbols are legitimate space savers in column and cut-in headings and in the body of tables, but not in titles (except for mathematical and chemical symbols). Standard abbreviations should be used if they exist; if they do not, the writer may devise abbreviations, explaining them in a note or key if necessary. Abbreviations must be consistent for all tables.

6.49 Symbols that cannot be made with the printer or typewriter should be inserted by hand, using a mechanical pen and black ink (see 7.27–32).

FOOTNOTES

6.50 Footnotes to a table are of four general kinds and should appear in this order: (1) source notes, (2) other general notes, (3) notes on specific parts of the table, and (4) notes on level of probability.

6.51 If data for a table are not the writer's own but are taken from another source, a source note should be included, introduced by the word *Source(s)*, in italics, followed by a colon:

Source: Michael H. Day, *Guide to Fossil Man*, 4th ed. (Chicago: University of Chicago Press, 1986), 291–304.

Any acknowledgment of permission to reproduce material is given in a source note:

Source: Reprinted, by permission of the publisher, from Ana-Maria Rizzuto, "Freud, God, the Devil, and the Theory of Object Representation," *International Review of Psycho-Analysis* 31 (1976): 165.

6.52 Other unnumbered notes, applying to the table as a whole, follow, introduced by the word *Note(s)* and a colon. These might include remarks on the reliability of the data presented or on how they were collected or handled; when practical, such notes should be gathered into one paragraph.

Notes: Since data were not available for all items on all individuals, there is some disparity in the totals. This table may be compared with table 14, which presents similar data for Cincinnati, Ohio.

6.53 For notes on specific parts of a table, superior letters (not italicized), beginning with *a* in each table, are usually employed as reference marks. They may be used on the column headings, on the stub items, and in the body of the table, but not on the table number or title. Any note applying to the number or title would be a general note and should be so treated. The reference marks come in whatever order the reader will find easiest to follow, normally beginning at the upper left and extending across the table and downward, row by row. The same mark may be used on two or more elements if the corresponding note applies to them.

6.54 Footnotes to tables must not be numbered in the same series as text notes. A new series of reference numbers or symbols is begun for each table.

6.55 For a table consisting only of words, superior numbers may be used as reference marks (though even here letters are quite usual); and for a table that includes mathematical or chemical equations, a series of arbitrary symbols may be used, because of the danger of mistaking superior letters or figures for exponents. The series is as follows:

```
* (asterisk or star), † (dagger), ‡ (double dagger),
§ (section mark), ‖ (parallels), # (number sign)
```

When more symbols are needed, these may be doubled and tripled in the same sequence:

```
**, ††, ‡‡, §§, ‖‖, ##, ***, †††, ‡‡‡, §§§, ‖‖‖, ###
```

6.56 In tables the reference marks—letters, numbers, or symbols—are conventionally placed in superior position before the notes themselves, not on the line as numbers may be in textual notes.

6.57 If a table contains values for which levels of probability are given, a fourth type of note is used, following the other specific notes. By convention, asterisks are used for these notes, both on the value in the body of the table and before the footnote. A single asterisk is used for the lowest level of probability, two for the next higher, and so on, with the specific levels given in the notes below:

```
* p < .05. ** p < .01. *** p < .001.
```

These short notes may be typed on the same line.

6.58 Footnotes are typed flush left below the body of the table. Double-space between items, single-space within. Leave a blank line between the table's closing rule and the first note. Three blank lines separate notes from any continuation of the text following a table.

RULING

6.59 Since some institutions specify that all tables must be ruled and others allow considerable latitude, it is advisable to consult the dissertation office. The following suggestions are for those who must make their own decisions.

6.60 Two-column tables are best left without any rules (sample 14.25). In general, all tables of more than two columns may carry vertical rules, but the fewer the better. It is permissible to omit the rules between columns covered by a spanner heading (see sample 14.27), provided the columns are not too close together. In sample 14.27, omitting rules between the columns is allowable; but in sample 14.28 the columns of figures are so close together that rules are important for ease of reading and therefore are not omitted. It is increasingly common to omit all vertical rules, even in very large tables, and this is acceptable if columns are appropriately spaced. Such tables are termed *open style* (see tables 5 and 6 above).

6.61 Each ruled table should have a horizontal rule at the top, above the column heads, and a horizontal rule at the end, above any notes. There are no vertical rules at the sides of a table.

6.62 Blank space should be left on all sides of a column heading. Never begin a heading on the line immediately below the rule, and never begin a rule on the same line as a heading (thus giving the effect of underlined words).

6.63 A horizontal rule may be typed above totals at the feet of columns, extending across the columns but not through the stub (see sample 14.27), or a blank line may be left. Subtotals, grand totals, means, and averages are similarly handled.

6.64 Horizontal rules can be made with the underscore key of the typewriter or computer. If the carriage of the typewriter will take the paper horizontally, all the rules can be typed, but vertical rules require special care if columns are only one or two spaces apart. Those using computer systems to prepare tables should consult a user's manual.

6.65 If vertical rules are made by hand, they should first be added to the typed or printed copy in very light, thin pencil and then retraced, using a mechanical pen with black ink and a ruler with an ink-absorbing edge. Press-apply type that offers a thin black adhesive line may also be placed along the pencil line. These materials will reproduce without appearing darker than the text or blurring (see also 7.30).

7 Illustrations

Line and Continuous-Tone Copy 7.2
Position 7.4
    Full-Page Illustrations 7.5
    Margins 7.7
    Two or More Illustrations on a Page 7.8
    Broadsides 7.9
    Legend 7.10
    Key or Scale 7.11
    Number and Legend 7.12
Figure Numbers and Legends 7.13
    Identifying Parts of an Illustration 7.16
    Credit Lines and Permissions 7.18
        Previously Published Material 7.21
        Original Material 7.23
Preparation 7.27
    Maps 7.33
    Computer Graphics 7.35
    Photographs 7.36
    Mounting 7.37
    Folding 7.44

7.1   Illustrative materials may consist of drawings, paintings, photographs, charts, graphs, and maps. Such illustrations are also called *figures*.

LINE AND CONTINUOUS-TONE COPY

7.2   Artwork containing only black and white, with no shading—a pen-and-ink drawing, for instance, or a bar chart—is known as *line copy.* Artwork that does contain shading—such as a painting, a wash drawing, or a photograph—is known as *continuous-tone copy* or, less accurately, *halftone copy.*

7.3   It is not within the scope of this manual to give advice on when to include illustrative materials or what types to use or, except in general terms, to give instructions on their presentation. These matters are fully treated in a number of specialized books. One of the best is Frances W. Zweifel's *Handbook of Biological Illustration.* Although it emphasizes biological illustrations, the treatment of many topics is equally helpful in other fields. Some general principles, however, do need to be summarized here.

POSITION

7.4   Illustrations, especially graphs and charts, should be placed as close as possible to their first references in the text. Like tables, they should be referred to by number so that their exact placement is flexible (see 6.13–17). There are sometimes sound reasons for grouping all the illustrations, if they are of one type, at the end of the paper or putting them in an appendix (see 1.39).

FULL-PAGE ILLUSTRATIONS

7.5   When illustrative materials are too large to be inserted in the text and consequently are placed on full pages by themselves, these pages are numbered consecutively with the text. It is not permissible to give them supplementary numbers (e.g., page 45a) after the text has been numbered. A folded map or chart is numbered in the center, at the top of the exposed fold (see also 7.44–46).

7.6   Illustrations placed together at the end of the paper follow the pagination of the text.

MARGINS

7.7   A margin of at least one inch should be allowed on all four edges of a page carrying illustrative material. More space is required on the left for papers that are to be bound, such as theses and dissertations. The number of the illustration and its caption or legend—everything but the page number—must fall within the margins (for margins when mounting material, see 7.41).

TWO OR MORE ILLUSTRATIONS ON A PAGE

7.8   Two or more figures may appear on the same page, each with its number and legend. Also, two or more related illustrations may be placed on the same page, the group as a whole given a single figure number, and the individual parts identified by letter (*a, b,* etc.). If space below the individual illustrations is not sufficient for separate legends, each one may simply be lettered, with the legends either grouped at the foot of the page or typed on the page opposite. In the latter instance, the page with the legends is turned over to precede and face the illustrations, so that the reader will see illustrations and legends together (see 6.23). The page facing the illustration is counted in the numbering of the paper, but no page number appears on it.

BROADSIDES

7.9   A wide illustration may be placed broadside on the page, with the top at the binding (left) side. The legend, with its number, should appear below the illustration so that it reads vertically up the page. The page number is in its normal position (see sample 14.24). This same arrangement may be used for a group of illustrations.

LEGEND

7.10   Some illustrations—maps in particular—carry typed or hand-lettered headings at the top or side. In such a case, only the spelled-out word *Figure* and the number are centered below the illustration.

KEY OR SCALE

7.11   A key or scale (of miles, inches, millimeters, etc.), if included, should be placed beside or within the illustration rather than below it.

NUMBER AND LEGEND

7.12   If the space below an illustration is not sufficient to carry the number and legend and still allow the one-inch margin at the bottom of the page, they may be placed within the illustration. If there is not enough space there, they may be placed on the page opposite (see 6.23 and 7.8).

FIGURE NUMBERS AND LEGENDS

7.13   Even if a paper contains several types of illustrations, such as maps, charts, diagrams, and graphs, it is desirable to label them all as figures and number them consecutively, using arabic numerals:

Fig. 43   Figure 2

7.14   A legend follows the number; this may be only a title, or caption:

Fig. 2. Block diagram of Fern Lake

The legend frequently consists of a sentence or more (not necessarily grammatically complete) of explanation, however. Here the punctuation and capitalization follow ordinary sentence style:

Fig. 9. Relation between number of buds or leaf scars, number of branches subsequently produced, and length of shoots. Small numbers identify multiple observations of same value.

7.15   The legend should be single-spaced and may run the width of the illustration. Short legends are centered.

IDENTIFYING PARTS OF AN ILLUSTRATION

7.16   Such terms as *top, bottom, left, right, above, below, left to right,* and *clockwise from left* are frequently used in legends to locate individual subjects in an illustration or parts of a composite. These are italicized or underlined and usually precede rather than follow the descriptive phrase:

Fig. 4. *Above left,* William Livingston; *right,* Henry Brockholst Livingston; *below left,* John Jay; *right,* Sarah Livingston Jay.

If a list follows the introductory tag, a colon rather than a comma is preferred:

Left to right: Dean Acheson, Harry Hopkins, President Roosevelt, Harold Ickes.

7.17 Letters of the alphabet, abbreviations, and symbols are all used as keys for identifying parts of a figure. When such a key is referred to in a legend, the form used there should reflect as closely as possible the form used in the figure itself. If capital letters are used in the figure, capitals should be used in the legend, and so on. In the legend, however, the key should be italicized or underlined, regardless of what is employed in the figure:

Fig. 5. Four types of Hawaiian fishhooks: a, barbed hook of tortoise shell; b, trolling hook with pearl shell lure and point of human bone; c, octopus lure with cowrie shell, stone sinker, and large bone hook; d, barbed hook of human thigh bone.

Fig. 6. Facial traits of (A) Propithecus verreauxi verreauxi and (B) Lemur catta, which vary from one individual to the next; ea, ear; ca, cap; cpl, capline; br, brow.

When symbols are used in a figure, using the symbols in the legend is easiest for the reader:

Fig. 7. Dependence of half-life on atomic weight for elements in the radium-uranium region: ○ = even α-emitters; ● = odd α-emitters; □ = isotopes capable of K-capture or β-decay.

If the symbols cannot be produced, they must be described:

Fig. 8. Dependence of half-life on atomic weight for elements in the radium-uranium region: open circles, even alpha-emitters; solid circles, odd alpha-emitters; open squares, isotopes capable of K-capture or beta-decay.

In the last example, note also that in a scientific context the names of the Greek letters may usually be substituted for the letters themselves.

CREDIT LINES AND PERMISSIONS

7.18 A brief statement of the source of the illustration is usually necessary or appropriate. The only significant exception is an illustration (chart, graph, drawing, photograph, etc.) created by the writer.

7.19   Illustrative material protected by copyright, whether published or unpublished, usually requires permission from the copyright owner before it can be reproduced even in a dissertation. It is the writer's responsibility to determine what is under copyright and obtain permission to use it (see 5.1).

7.20   The credit line may run at the end of the legend, usually in parentheses, or the pertinent facts may be worked into the legend. If most or all of the illustrations are from a single source, that fact may be stated in the preface or acknowledgments.

PREVIOUSLY PUBLISHED MATERIAL

7.21   There is no fixed style for such credit lines, but they should be consistent and, for a work of book length, should include a page number, figure number, or the like. A short form is appropriate if the work the illustration has been taken from is listed in the bibliography or reference list. The person who grants permission to reproduce the illustration may, however, specify a certain form of credit including the full facts of publication and even a copyright notice.

[*a kinship diagram*]

```
Reprinted, by permission, from Wagner, Curse of Souw,
82.
```

[*a portrait engraving*]

```
From a drawing by J. Webber for Cook's Voyage to the
Pacific Ocean, 1776-1780, reprinted, by permission of
the writer, from Edwin H. Bryan, Jr., Ancient Hawaiian
Life (Honolulu, 1938), 10.
```

[*a photograph*]

```
Reprinted, by permission, from Alison Jolly, Lemur
Behavior, pl. 6. Photograph by C. H. Fraser Rowell.
© 1966 by The University of Chicago.
```

7.22   Illustrations may be reproduced from published works without seeking permission if the work is in the public domain: that is, if it was never in copyright (as is true of most publications of the United States government) or if the copyright has run full term and lapsed. Even though permission is not required, it is good policy to use a credit line out of deference to the reader as well as the creator of the material.

Illustration by Joseph Pennell for Henry James, *English Hours* (Boston, 1905), facing p. 82.

Reprinted from John D. Shortridge, *Italian Harpsichord Building in the Sixteenth and Seventeenth Centuries,* U.S. National Museum Bulletin 225 (Washington, D.C., n.d.).

ORIGINAL MATERIAL

7.23 Although illustrations that are the writer's own work do not need credit lines, this does not mean credit lines should not be used if there is some reason for them. If, for example, all but a few of the illustrations are from one source and this source is acknowledged in the preliminaries, it would be appropriate to place under a photograph taken by the writer a line reading:

Photograph by the author

or

Photo by author

Somewhat different is the case of material commissioned by the writer, usually maps, photographs, or drawings. Here professional courtesy dictates mention of the creator either in the preliminaries or below each piece, where the credit line might read as follows:

Map by Gerald F. Pyle
Photograph by James L. Ballard
Drawing by Joseph E. Alderfer

If a map or drawing is signed and the signature is reproduced, nothing further is needed.

7.24 For material that the writer has obtained free of charge and without restrictions on its use, a credit line is seldom legally required but usually is appended nonetheless. In such credit lines it is appropriate to use the word *courtesy:*

Photograph courtesy of Ford Motor Company

or

Courtesy of Ford Motor Co.

If the name of the photographer is well known, or if the supplier of the print requests it, the photographer's name may also be given:

```
Photograph by Henri Cartier-Bresson, courtesy of the
Museum of Modern Art
```

7.25 Material obtained from a commercial agency—photographs and reproductions of prints, drawings, paintings, and the like—usually requires a credit line. The contract or bill of sale will specify what is expected. Typical credits:

```
Woodcut from Historical Pictures Service, Chicago

Photograph from Wide World Photos
```

7.26 Sometimes a writer does not directly reproduce another's material but nonetheless is indebted to that person. The writer may, for example, use data from a table in a book to construct a chart, or revise another's graph with fresh data, or redraw a figure with or without significant changes. In such situations, although the writer's material is technically original, a credit line is in order. Again, there is no set form. Thus for a chart based on a table in another work, the credit line might read:

```
Data from John F. Witte, Democracy, Authority, and
Alienation in Work (Chicago: University of Chicago
Press, 1980), table 10
```

If the book is listed fully elsewhere in the paper, the citation could be:

```
Data from Witte, Democracy, Authority, and Alienation
in Work, table 10
```

   or

```
Data from Witte 1980, table 10
```

PREPARATION

7.27 Since many colleges and universities have graphic arts departments that prepare dissertation- and publication-quality illustrations, only professional artwork now has a place in theses and dissertations and the articles for professional journals or other scholarly publications that are based on them.

7.28 In the absence of such services or if one is preparing a term paper, for example, artwork can be rendered more professionally by using the materials graphic artists now use. Most are available at art supply stores.

7.29 Color should not be used in a thesis or dissertation for a university that requires microfilm reproduction of such papers.

111

Although color may be necessary in research papers on art, medical, or other color-related topics, press-apply tones can be substituted in most cases. When microfilm reproduction is not required, color may be used for line drawings if suitable photo-duplicating equipment is available, and color photographs may be included when the colors in them are absolutely necessary to the paper. When color or black-and-white photographs are required, they may be mounted individually in each copy of the paper or developed on lightweight photographic paper, leaving a suitable white margin.

7.30 To design linear graphs, charts, and the like, use graph paper with lines that disappear in photoduplication. Lightly draw in all lines first, using a mechanical pencil. Then go over these lightly penciled lines with a mechanical pen using black ink, resting it against a double-ink edge (to prevent blurring of lines). Or place a press-apply line over the lightly penciled one. Press-apply tones and lines are available in many varieties. They do not smudge or blur, and they can easily be moved before they are burnished into place.

7.31 Add letters, symbols, curves, and numbers only after the inked or adhesive lines (and tones, if any) are in place. Templates and adjustable curves may be used with a mechanical pen and black ink, or one of the many press-apply forms of lettering, numbers, and symbols may be used. Templates and press-apply forms are available in many typefaces and a variety of point sizes. Illustrations created using these products must be photo-copied before they are inserted in the paper (see 13.37).

7.32 It is usually best to render a drawing larger than it will be on the page and then reduce it onto acid-free paper (see 13.35 for a description of this paper stock) through either photographic or photoduplicating methods, especially when fine detail must be shown in the illustration.

MAPS

7.33 Many kinds of maps are available ready-made, and some are satisfactory with no additions except page and figure numbers and possibly a legend (see sample 14.24). Some may be used as base maps, with cross-hatching, outlining of specific areas, and figures or letters superimposed. Unless cross-hatching covers only a small area, handwork should not be attempted. Press-apply tones are available in many designs, but illustrations made with them must be photocopied before being inserted in the paper (see 13.37).

7.34   Although maps are frequently executed entirely by hand, it is now possible to generate them by computer (see Mark Monmonier, *Mapping It Out*). In the fields of geography and geology, where knowledge of maps and mapmaking is an important aspect of the student's training, handmade or computer-generated maps are likely to be required in theses and dissertations.

COMPUTER GRAPHICS

7.35   Computer software is available that converts raw laboratory data into conventional graphics with corresponding legends, and some programs can produce graphs with labeled axes, interval marks, and symbols as well as curves or histograms. Before using such a program to produce an illustration, consult either the user's manual or a computer adviser so that the artwork will have the proper dimensions for the paper or for photoduplication, microfilming, and any reduction needed to bring it within the specifications set by a department or discipline. Continuous-tone illustrations (color and black-and-white), animations, and three-dimensional subjects may also be technically feasible on computers, and such illustrations should be acceptable if they meet the requirements for size and quality of reproduction specified by the institution. See chapter 13 for discussions of computer graphics (13.21–23), printing (13.24–30), and photoduplicating (13.36–37).

PHOTOGRAPHS

7.36   Photographs should be finished 6 by 9 inches or smaller and mounted one or more to a page on full-size (8½-by-11-inch) sheets of single-weight acid-free paper. Matte-surface photographs are preferable to glossy prints, although the latter are sharper and therefore a better choice where minute detail must be shown.

MOUNTING

7.37   Color photographs or other color reproductions are the only
illustrations that should be mounted within a finished thesis or
dissertation (but see 7.29). Black-and-white photographs (except where extremely accurate reproduction of detail is
needed), artwork, and color line drawings should all be reproduced through one of several means of photoduplication. For
example, photographs can be reproduced on single-weight
8½-by-11-inch acid-free paper, allowing for a suitable white
margin, using a screening process readily available in graphic
arts departments on many campuses.

7.38   Dry-mounting tissue is the most satisfactory adhesive for
mounting illustrations. Properly applied—and correct application is most important—the mounts will remain firm for many
years without causing deterioration of the illustrations. The tissue is available in sheets or in rolls, accompanied by complete
directions for its use, and can be purchased from photographic
and art supply stores.

7.39   Although dry mounting is preferred for illustrations designed
for long-term use, some glue sticks or double-faced tapes are
reasonably satisfactory. Some institutions will not accept their
use, however, so check with the dissertation office.

7.40   Before doing the final mountings, it is wise to experiment with
positioning, using special tape that is only slightly adhesive
and will not mar the illustration.

7.41   Whatever adhesive is used, the area of the paper to be covered
by the illustration should be marked before the mounts are put
in place by drawing a very light pencil line at the top or by
placing a dot at each upper corner. The illustration, or the
composite of illustrations, should be centered on the page.
Centering, in this connection, assumes a slightly wider margin
at the bottom of the sheet than at the top, and a half inch wider
margin at the left than at the right (to accommodate binding).

7.42   When using dry-mounting tissue, as each page of material is
mounted, set it aside to dry for a few minutes (follow the directions precisely), then put pieces of plain paper between the
sheets and place them under a weight for several hours.

7.43 Be sure to allow sufficient time for mounting illustrations. The inexperienced person is likely to underestimate the time required to do this work satisfactorily.

FOLDING

7.44 Illustrations larger than the normal page size usually may be reduced photographically. If reduction is not feasible, as in the case of large maps, for example, the material may be folded, provided the institution the paper is prepared for does not prohibit it.

7.45 To fold, work first from right to left, making the first crease no more than 7$\frac{1}{2}$ inches from the left side of the sheet, which should have a 1$\frac{1}{2}$-inch margin. If a second fold is necessary, carry the right-hand portion of the sheet back to the right, making the second crease no more than 6$\frac{1}{2}$ inches to the left of the first. Additional folds, if required, should be parallel to the first two. If the folding is done as directed, the folds at the left will not be caught in the stitching nor those at the right sheared off during trimming.

7.46 Folding in more than one direction should be avoided, but when such folding is necessary, the sheet should first be folded from bottom to top, making the first fold no more than 10 inches from the top of the sheet. When this first fold has been made, unfold the sheet and cut a strip 1 inch wide from the left side, starting at the bottom and continuing up to the fold. Removing this strip prevents the free portion of the sheet from being caught in the stitching. The sheet may then be refolded and folded from right to left as directed above.

8   Notes

Method of Citation 8.1
Uses of Notes 8.3
Note Numbers 8.7
Position of Notes 8.15
Abbreviations in Notes 8.17
Reference Notes 8.21
Books 8.23
   First, Full Reference 8.23
      Name of Author 8.26
      Title of Work 8.37
      Name of Editor, Translator, or Compiler 8.40
      Name of Author of Preface, Foreword, or Introduction
         8.43
      Edition 8.44
         Numbered Edition 8.45
         Reprint Edition 8.46
         Paperback Edition 8.47
         Named Edition 8.48
      Name of Series 8.49
      Facts of Publication 8.51
         Place of Publication 8.52
         Name of Publishing Agency 8.57
         Date of Publication 8.67
      Page References 8.70
      Multivolume Works 8.74
   Subsequent References 8.84
      Ibid. 8.85
      Shortened References 8.88
         Method A 8.90
         Method B 8.91
         Short Titles 8.94

Periodicals 8.97
　　Journals 8.99
　　Magazines 8.104
　　Newspapers 8.105
　　Subsequent References 8.111
Special Forms 8.112
　　Articles in Encyclopedias and Dictionaries 8.112
　　Novels, Plays, and Poems 8.113
　　　　Novels 8.113
　　　　Plays and Long Poems 8.114
　　　　Short Poems 8.116
　　Reviews 8.117
　　Interviews 8.118
　　Greek and Latin Classical Works 8.119
　　Medieval Works 8.128
　　Scriptural References 8.129
　　Unpublished Material 8.130
　　Legal Citations 8.133
　　Public Documents 8.136
　　Microform Editions 8.137
　　Material Obtained through Loose-Leaf or Information
　　　　Services 8.139
　　Computer Programs 8.140
　　Electronic Documents 8.141
　　Musical Scores 8.142
　　Musical Compositions 8.143
　　Sound Recordings 8.144
　　Videorecordings 8.145
　　Performances 8.146
　　Works of Art 8.147
　　Citations Taken from Secondary Sources 8.148
Content Notes 8.149
Cross-References 8.150

METHOD OF CITATION

8.1　Writers of term papers, theses, and dissertations should first of all determine whether a particular method of documentation is required by their academic department or discipline. If a style is specified, the writer should follow an authoritative manual within that field (see the bibliography at the back of this manual). In the natural and social sciences, the use of parenthetical references and a reference list is generally recommended. This method of documentation, often called the author-date style, is discussed in chapter 10. The Modern Language Association has its own guidelines for a parenthetical documentation style, although the system employing notes and a bibliography has long been preferred in most areas of the humanities. This second, or humanities, style of documentation is described here.

8.2   Using footnotes rather than endnotes or parenthetical references allows a paper to be read from beginning to end on microfilm without searching for a reference in the back matter. For theses and dissertations that are held and distributed on microfilm, particularly those in the humanities, where footnotes have traditionally been used, footnotes and a bibliography are preferred. Since endnotes are not acceptable in some academic departments and institutions, the writer should ascertain the requirements before using this form of documentation. For the rules governing bibliographical style, see chapter 9; for examples of notes and corresponding bibliographica entries, see chapter 11. Guidelines for the layout of footnotes, bibliographies, and endnotes are also included in chapter 14.

USES OF NOTES

8.3   Notes have four main uses: (*a*) to cite the authority for statements in text—specific facts or opinions as well as exact quotations; (*b*) to make cross-references; (*c*) to make incidental comments on, to amplify, or to qualify textual discussion—in short, to provide a place for material the writer deems worthwhile to include but that might interrupt the flow of thought if introduced into the text; and (*d*) to make acknowledgments. Notes, then, are of two kinds: *reference* (*a* and *b*) and *content* (*c* and *d*). A content note may also include one or more references (see 8.149). Descriptions and examples of note form are given in the following pages.

8.4   Tables, outlines, lists, letters, and the like that are not immediately relevant to the text are best placed in an appendix and referred to in the text by a simple content footnote:

```
⁵The member banks and their contributors are
listed in appendix 3.
```

In a paper using endnotes or parenthetical references, references to the materials above should be placed in parentheses in the text, so that the reader does not have to consult two parts of the back matter to find a source:

```
Auditors traced this error to the member banks and
their contributors (see appendix 3).
```

8.5   If a block quotation (see 5.4) contains note references from the original source, the corresponding notes should be placed beneath the quotation, not among the notes belonging to the paper itself. An eight-space rule (made by underscoring) separates the note or notes from the quotation. The reference index—whether number or symbol—and the form of the note should follow exactly the style of the original material:

```
Given the course of events, they might all have said,
along with Bataille himself:

        My tension, in a sense, resembles a great
    welling up of laughter, it is not unlike the burning
    passions of Sade's heroes, and yet, it is close to
    that of the martyrs, or of the saints.²³
```

```
        ²³"Ma tension ressemble, en un sens, à une folle
    envie de rire, elle diffère peu des passions dont
    brûlent les héros de Sade, et pourtant, elle est
    proche de celle des martyrs ou des saints" (Sur
    Nietzsche, 12).⁸
```

A note reference at the end of the whole quotation (like the reference [8] above) is numbered in sequence with the rest of the notes in the paper. If the writer of the paper adds note references within the block quotation—to identify persons mentioned, for example, or to translate words or passages in a foreign language—those references are also numbered in sequence with the paper's notes. The corresponding notes are placed at the bottom of the page, or at the end of the paper if endnotes are being used.

8.6   Unless they are short and simple, tables, outlines, lists, letters, and the like should not be placed in notes.

NOTE NUMBERS

8.7 The place in the text where a note is introduced, whether footnote or endnote, reference or content, is marked with an arabic numeral typed slightly above the line (superscript).

8.8 Most computer systems and many typewriters can elevate characters a uniform half space above the line of text, and some can make them smaller. Never elevate note numbers a full space. If the computer system used cannot produce superscript numbers, leave space in the text and add them using a typewriter with a compatible typeface.

8.9 Do not put a period after a superscript note number or embellish it with parentheses, brackets, or slash marks. The note reference follows any punctuation mark except the dash, which it precedes, and goes outside a closing parenthesis.

8.10 Note numbers preceding the footnotes themselves are preferably typed on the line, followed by a period (see 14.14). If the computer system used generates footnotes with superscript numbers, however, that is also acceptable. On-line numerals should always be used with endnotes. Both styles are illustrated here and in other chapters. The first line of the footnote is indented the same amount as paragraph openings in the text.

8.11 The note reference should follow the passage it refers to. If the passage is an exact quotation, the note number comes at the end of it, not after the author's name or at the end of the textual matter introducing the quotation. If possible, a note number should come at the end of a sentence, or at least at the end of a clause.

8.12 Note numbers must follow one another in numerical order, beginning with 1. Numbering starts over at the beginning of each chapter. In papers that are not divided into chapters, the numbers will run continuously throughout. Care must be taken to ensure that the final sequence is correct. If checking the manuscript reveals that a note has been omitted or that one should be deleted, the notes must be renumbered from that point to the end of the chapter or paper. Inserting a note numbered, for example, *2a* is not permissible, nor is omitting a number.

8.13 Some computer systems number notes automatically and will renumber if a note is added or deleted (see 13.17).

8.14 Double numbers (such as [1,2]) may not be used except in scientific fields where this practice is acceptable (see 10.33). Consult an authoritative manual within the discipline for guidelines (see the bibliography at the end of this manual).

POSITION OF NOTES

8.15 Notes should be placed in numerical order at the foot of the page (footnotes) below a short rule, or *separator* (see 14.13), or at the end of the paper if endnotes are used (but see 8.2). A footnote must begin on the page where it is referenced, though a long note may extend to the bottom of the next page (see sample 14.36). Notes may be single-spaced, with a blank line between them.

8.16 Time and space can be saved and the appearance of the page improved by reducing the number of note references in the text. In a single paragraph containing several quotations, for example, a reference number following the last quotation will permit them all to be cited in one note. For example:

```
The means by which the traditional Western composers
have attempted to communicate with their audience have
been discussed at length by Eduard Hanslick,[2] Heinrich
Schenker,[3] Suzanne Langer,[4] and Leonard Meyer,[5] to name
but a few.
```

Could be replaced by:

```
The means by which the traditional Western composers
have attempted to communicate with their audience have
been discussed at length by Eduard Hanslick, Heinrich
Schenker, Suzanne Langer, and Leonard Meyer, to name
but a few.[2]
```

The single footnote would then read:

```
     2. Eduard Hanslick, The Beautiful in Music, trans.
G. Cohen (New York: Novello, Ewer, 1891); Heinrich
Schenker, Der freie Satz, trans. and ed. T. H. Kreuger
(Ann Arbor: University Microfilms, 1960), pub. no. 60-
1558; Suzanne Langer, Philosophy in a New Key (New
York: Mentor, 1959); Leonard B. Meyer, Emotion and
Meaning in Music (Chicago: University of Chicago Press,
1956), and idem, Music, the Arts, and Ideas (Chicago:
University of Chicago Press, 1967).
```

ABBREVIATIONS IN NOTES

8.17   Except in scientific and technical writing, few abbreviations are permissible in text (see 2.1), but in notes, bibliographies, reference lists, tabular matter, and some kinds of illustrative matter abbreviations are normally preferred. Abbreviations commonly found in these parts of a paper are listed in 2.18 and 2.23–26.

8.18   Abbreviations for parts of a written work (*vol., pt., chap.,* etc.) should never be used unless followed or preceded by a number (*vol. 2, 4 vols., pt. 1, chap. 10,* etc.). When used without numbers, these words should be spelled out.

8.19   Titles of journals, dictionaries, and other sources used frequently in a paper may be abbreviated by the initials of the words of their titles, without spaces or periods between the letters. Such abbreviations are permissible in notes but not in bibliographical entries or some kinds of reference lists (see also 10.30 and 10.34).

American Historical Review	AHR
Nouvelle Revue Française	NRF
Dictionary of National Biography	DNB
Oxford English Dictionary	OED

Journals that have initials as actual titles should be so cited in bibliographies and reference lists as well as in notes:

PMLA   MLN   ELN

8.20   A writer who must refer frequently to the same work may devise a short form to be used after the first, full reference, but complete words from the work's title should be used rather than an acronym or initials only.

Pagan Mysteries of the Renaissance   Pagan Mysteries

See also 8.94–96.

REFERENCE NOTES

8.21   Notes that contain references, or citations, to sources are called reference, or documentation, notes. Although such notes may also contain some discussion or amplification of the text (see 8.149), our concern here is with the form of the citations. Chapter 9 will present the preferred forms for bibliography entries corresponding to citations in notes. Samples of reference notes and corresponding bibliography entries are provided in chapters 11 and 12. For the layout of notes on the page, see 14.13–17 for directions and 14.35 and 14.36 for samples.

8.22 The first time a work is mentioned in a note, the entry should be in complete form; that is, it should include not only the author's full name, the title of the work, and the specific reference (volume, if any, and page number), but the facts of publication as well. For a book the source of information is the title page and copyright page; for a periodical it is the cover and the article itself. Once a work has been cited in full, subsequent references to it should be in shortened form. These forms are fully discussed and illustrated in 8.84–96.

BOOKS

FIRST, FULL REFERENCE

8.23 With some exceptions, such as references to legal, classical, and biblical works and to certain classes of public documents (see chapter 12), information in notes citing a published work for the first time is given in the sequence indicated in 8.24–25.

8.24 For a book, the first, full reference should include the following information in the order shown:

> Name of author(s)
> Title and (if any) subtitle
> Name of editor, compiler, or translator, if any
> Number or name of edition, if other than the first
> Name of series in which book appears, if any, with volume or number in the series
> Facts of publication, consisting of
>> Place of publication
>> Name of publishing agency
>> Date of publication
> Page number(s) of the specific citation

In note references, the elements above are separated by commas or, in the case of the facts of publication, parentheses.

Note that the comma following the book title or the designation of edition is replaced by the opening parenthesis of the publication facts. The comma following the publication facts and preceding the page reference is retained, however. In bibliographies, as is shown in chapter 9, the elements are separated by periods.

8.25   The first, full reference to a preface, foreword, introduction, chapter, appendix, or similar part of a book begins with the name of the author of that part. This is followed by the title of the part and then the rest of the items listed in 8.24. The author or editor of the book itself is given only if different from the author of the part.

> [1]Arthur Danhurst, introduction to *Calculating the Incalculable,* by Samuel Ifferson (Minneapolis: Naughtinton Press, 1994), 2-4.

> [2]Samuel Ifferson, preface to *Calculating the Incalculable,* . . .

> [3]Samuel Ifferson, "Basic Methods," in *Calculating* . . .

> [4]Norwald Torrington, "Following the Path to the Left," in *Whither Tomorrow?* ed. Montgomery Abelson (Tulsa: Wizmer Bros., 1994).

Note that in the first and second examples the preposition *to* is added before the title of the book as a whole; but if the part cited is a chapter, as in the third example, *in* is used. The fourth example illustrates the form used when the author of a chapter is not the author of the book. See also 8.43.

NAME OF AUTHOR

8.26   Whether or not it appears close to the citation in the text, the author's name must be given in the reference. Present the name in normal order—given name before family name (Robert John Blank, for example)—and follow with a comma. The name should appear as it does on the title page or in a byline. Except for well-known authors who habitually use only the initials of their given names (e.g., T. S. Eliot, D. H. Lawrence, J. B. S. Haldane, W. B. Yeats), initials only should not be used if the author's given names are known.

8.27   If the title page, or the byline at the head of a chapter or article, gives a pseudonym known to be that of a certain author, give the pseudonym only. The pseudonym followed by the author's real name in brackets appears in bibliographies and reference lists (see 11.9). Such familiar pseudonyms as Anatole France, George Eliot, and Mark Twain, however, may be used throughout a paper in place of the real name.

8.28   If a pseudonym is labeled as such on the title page or in the byline, the abbreviation *pseud.* is enclosed in parentheses and placed after the pseudonym: Helen Delay (pseud.).

8.29   If pseudonymity is not indicated on the title page or in the byline but is nevertheless an established fact, the abbreviation *pseud.* may be placed in brackets after the pseudonym, or the author's real name, if known, may be placed in brackets after it.

8.30   If the title page or byline gives no author's name, or if it designates the work as anonymous, and if in either case the authorship has been definitely established, the author's name, in brackets, may be placed before the title:

> 1. [Elizabeth DeLor], *Revelation in Babylon* (Portland, Ore.: McCumber and Swillsworth, 1994).

Using *anonymous* in place of the name of an author is not recommended. If the authorship is not reliably established, the note reference should begin with the title of the work.

8.31   For a work by two or by three authors, give the full names in normal order, separating the names of two authors with *and* and those of three authors with commas, the last comma followed by *and:*

> ¹Mary Lyon, Bryce Lyon, and Henry S. Lucas, *The Wardrobe Book of William de Norwell, 12 July 1338 to 27 May 1340,* with the collaboration of Jean de Sturler (Brussels: Commission Royale d'Histoire de Belgique, 1983), 175.

> ²Dana Carleton Munro and Raymond James Sontag, *The Middle Ages, 395-1500,* rev. ed., Century Historical Series (New York and London: Century, 1928), 69.

8.32   If a work has more than three authors, it is usual to cite in the note (but not in the bibliography or reference list) only the name of the author given first on the title page and to follow it with *et al.* or its English equivalent, *and others.* Whichever one you choose, follow the same style throughout the paper. No comma comes between the author's name and *et al.* A period always follows *al.* (see also 11.6)

> 2. Martin Greenberger et al., eds., *Networks for Research and Education: Sharing of Computer Information Resources Nationwide* (Cambridge: MIT Press, 1974), 54.

8.33 For coauthors with the same family name, cite each name in full in the first reference—Sidney Webb and Beatrice Webb, not Sidney and Beatrice Webb. In later references write "Webb and Webb," not "the Webbs" (see 11.4).

8.34 Even though a title page or byline may include a title such as doctor, professor, or president or give a scholastic degree or official position, all such designations should be omitted except in rare instances where they would have significance for the subject of the paper:

> ¹Leon R. Kass, M.D., *Toward a More Natural Science: Biology and Human Affairs* (New York: Free Press, 1985), 252.

8.35 The "author" may be a corporate body—a country, state, city, legislative body, institution, society, business firm, committee, or the like (see example 11.10).

8.36 Some works—compilations, anthologies—are produced by editors or compilers, whose names are given in place of authors' names and are followed by the abbreviation *ed.* (*eds.*) or *comp.* (*comps.*).

> 1. Max Komatose, Ira Sneed, and Sarah Swidher, eds., *Ensemble Acting in the Off-Loop Theaters of Chicago* (Toledo: Wright-Smart Press, 1995), 193.

See also example 11.11.

TITLE OF WORK

8.37 Enter the full title (and subtitle, if any) of a book as it appears on the title page. See 8.39 for instructions on punctuating titles and subtitles that are distinguished on the title page by size and style of type rather than by punctuation. Enter the title of a chapter or other part of a book as it appears in the work. Adhere to any peculiarities of spelling and punctuation within titles, but in notes capitalize the titles of all works headline style (see 4.6–8), whether they are published or unpublished.

8.38   Italicize or underline the title of a whole published work, such as a book or periodical. Enclose in quotation marks the title of a chapter in a book. Place a comma after the title of a book unless it is followed immediately by parentheses enclosing the facts of publication, in which case the comma follows the final parenthesis (see 11.3).

> ²E. J. Clegg and J. P. Garlick, eds., *Disease and Urbanization,* Symposia of the Society for the Study of Human Biology, vol. 20 (Atlantic Highlands, N.J.: Humanities Press International, 1980), 16.

> ³Virgil Thomson, "Cage and the Collage of Noises," in *American Music since 1910* (New York: Holt, Rinehart, and Winston, 1971), 25.

8.39   Since display headings on title pages and articles are frequently set in two or more lines, with punctuation omitted at the end of each line, it is often necessary to add punctuation to a title as written out in text, notes, reference lists, or bibliographies. Commas must sometimes be added, particularly before dates, but the most common need is for a colon between main title and subtitle:

> *The Early Growth of Logic in the Child*
> *Classification and Seriation*

When the title and subtitle are referred to, they appear as follows:

> *The Early Growth of Logic in the Child: Classification and Seriation*

NAME OF EDITOR, TRANSLATOR, OR COMPILER

8.40   If in addition to the name of an author the title page contains that of an editor, translator, or compiler, that name follows the title, preceded by a comma and the appropriate abbreviation: *ed.* or *trans.* or *comp.* In this case the abbreviation stands for *edited by* or *translated by* or *compiled by* and thus is never in the plural:

> 1. Edward Chiera, *They Wrote on Clay,* ed. George G. Cameron (Chicago: University of Chicago Press, 1938), 42.

> 2. John Stuart Mill, *Autobiography and Literary Essays,* ed. John M. Robson and Jack Stillinger (Toronto: University of Toronto Press, 1980), 15.

8.41   A work may have both an editor and a translator as well as an author, and the same person may be both editor and translator:

> ¹August von Haxthausen, *Studies on the Interior of Russia,* ed. S. Frederick Starr, trans. Eleanore L. M. Schmidt (Chicago: University of Chicago Press, 1972), 47.

> ²Helmut Thielicke, *Man in God's World,* trans. and ed. John W. Doberstein (New York: Harper & Row, 1963), 43.

8.42   Similar in style is the entry for an edited or translated work in which the author's name is included in the title. Here the author's name as the first item of information is omitted, although it might properly be inserted even though it is not on the title page:

> 1. *The Works of Shakespear,* ed. Alexander Pope (London: printed for Jacob Tonson in the Strand, 1725), 6:20.

> *or*

> 1. William Shakespeare, *The Works of Shakespear,* ed. Alexander Pope (London: printed for Jacob Tonson in the Strand, 1725), 6:20.

Although the foregoing arrangement, which gives the editor's name following the title, is most commonly used for this kind of work, in a paper dealing primarily with the work of Pope it would be permissible to give his name first, followed by *ed.*:

> 1. Alexander Pope, ed., *The Works of Shakespear* (London: printed for Jacob Tonson in the Strand, 1725), 6:20.

A bibliographical entry begins with the author's name even if the name is also in the title (see 11.13).

NAME OF AUTHOR OF PREFACE, FOREWORD, OR INTRODUCTION

8.43   It is sometimes desirable to include in the source citation a reference to a preface, foreword, or introduction written by someone other than the author of the book itself. Such information is normally added between the title and the facts of publication, preceded by a comma:

¹Dag Hammarskjöld, *Markings,* with a foreword by W. H. Auden (New York: Alfred A. Knopf, 1964), 38.

If the citation is primarily to such a preface, foreword, or introduction, however, that information precedes the citation to the book itself (see also 8.25):

¹W. H. Auden, foreword to *Markings,* by Dag Hammarskjöld (New York: Alfred A. Knopf, 1964), ix.

or

¹W. H. Auden, foreword to Dag Hammarskjöld, *Markings* (New York: Alfred A. Knopf, 1964), ix.

Note that there are two ways of including the author of the book from which the foreword is cited.

EDITION

8.44   Information concerning the edition is required if the work cited is not the first edition. The information is frequently printed on the title page, but it is often found on the copyright page (the reverse of the title page). Besides numbered editions, there are reprint editions, paperback editions, and named editions.

8.45   *Numbered edition.* Although new editions are usually numbered, they may be designated on the title page merely as New Edition or New Revised Edition (abbreviated in notes, bibliographies, and reference lists as rev. ed., new rev. ed., etc.) and so on. Also found are Second Edition, Revised (2d ed., rev.); Revised Second Edition (rev. 2d ed.); Third Edition, Revised and Enlarged (3d ed., rev. and enl.); Revised Edition in One Volume (rev. ed. in 1 vol.); Fourth Edition, Revised by John Doe (4th ed., rev. John Doe); and so forth:

5. William Garzke Jr. and Robert O. Dulin Jr., *Battleships: Axis Battleships in World War II,* 3d ed., Battleship Series, vol. 3 (Annapolis, Md.: Naval Institute Press, 1985), 379.

6. Richard Ellmann, *James Joyce,* new and rev. ed. (New York: Oxford University Press, 1982), 705.

8.46   *Reprint edition.* Works that are out of print may be reissued in special reprint editions. Since the pagination is often different from that of the original, it is important to note which edition is being cited. Notes, reference lists, and bibliographies should include the reprint information and also give the date of the original publication and if possible the original publisher (see 11.19):

> [1]Gunnar Myrdal, *Population: A Problem for Democracy* (Cambridge: Harvard University Press, 1940; reprint, Gloucester, Mass.: Peter Smith, 1956), 9.

It is not necessary to note a new printing—for example, fourth impression—by the original publisher.

8.47 *Paperback edition.* Not all paperback editions are reprints, but when they are, they should be treated as reprints, giving original publication data as well as reprint data. A book published originally as a paperback should be listed like any other book, except that the name of the press or series may identify it as a paperback (see 11.20):

> 4. Mary Wollstonecraft Shelley, *Frankenstein, or The Modern Prometheus: The 1818 Text,* ed. James Reiger (Indianapolis: Bobbs-Merrill, 1974; Chicago: University of Chicago Press, Phoenix Books, 1982), 37.
>
> 5. Leon F. Litwack, *North of Slavery: The Negro in the Free States, 1790-1860* (Chicago: University of Chicago Press, 1961; Phoenix Books, 1965), 65.
>
> 6. Howard P. Segal, *Technological Utopianism in American Culture* (Chicago: University of Chicago Press, Chicago Original Paperback, 1985), 31.

8.48 *Named edition.* Many classics are found in named editions. When they are used in references, they should be specified:

> [9]Blaise Pascal, *Pensées and the Provincial Letters,* Modern Library ed. (New York: Random House, 1941), 418.

The title pages of some named editions do not give the name of the publisher. If only city and date can be given, they are separated by a comma.

NAME OF SERIES

8.49 Books and pamphlets are sometimes published as parts of named series (e.g., Oxford English Monographs, Yale Studies in Political Science, Monographs of the Society for Research in Child Development), which are sponsored by publishers, institutions—especially universities and graduate schools—government agencies, learned societies, commercial and industrial firms, and so on. Although a series bears some resemblance to a periodical publication and to a multivolume work, there are important differences stemming from individual plans of publication—differences that are reflected in the particular style of reference appropriate to each.

8.50 The publication of a series is an ongoing project of its sponsors, whose purpose is to issue from time to time books or pamphlets by different writers on topics that may range rather widely over a specific field or discipline or area of interest. Many series are numbered; the citation of a particular work in a numbered series should include the volume number (or issue number) after the name of the series. Note that the volume number here applies to the series and the page number to the book; therefore the citation differs from that for a multivolume work (see 8.74). Note also that although the title of the work is italicized, the name of the series is not, nor is it put in quotation marks:

> 1. Luli Callinicos, *Workers on the Rand: Factories, Townships, and Popular Culture, 1886-1942,* A People's History of South Africa, vol. 2 (Athens: Ohio University Press, 1985), 48.

> 2. Kenneth M. Setton, *The Papacy and the Levant 1204-1571,* vol. 1, *The Thirteenth and Fourteenth Centuries,* Memoirs of the American Philosophical Society, no. 114 (Philadelphia: American Philosophical Society, 1976), 398-400.

> 3. Leonard L. Watkins, *Commercial Banking Reform in the United States,* Michigan Business Studies, vol. 6, no. 5 (Ann Arbor: University of Michigan, 1938), 464.

FACTS OF PUBLICATION

8.51 As listed in 8.24, the facts of publication include place (city), publishing agency, and date. They appear in notes as follows:

> (London: Hogarth Press, 1964)

These facts are given for printed books, monographs, and pamphlets and for published works that are mimeographed, photocopied, microfilmed, or otherwise reproduced. But note the following exceptions:

1. Citations of biblical, classical, and medieval works omit all facts of publication (see 8.119–29).

2. Citations of legal works and some public documents usually omit all but the date (see 8.133–35).

3. Citations of dictionaries, general encyclopedias, and atlases omit all but the edition and date (see 8.112).

4. In certain disciplines, citations omit name of publisher (see 8.66 and 10.34).

5. Citations of periodicals generally omit all but the date (8.97–98).

8.52   *Place of publication.* If the names of two or more cities appear under the publisher's imprint, the first name is normally all that is needed in the reference, though it is permissible to use both. Do not add cities that do not appear on the title page (see 8.55).

8.53   If the city is not widely known, give the state as well, using the standard abbreviation, such as "Glenview, Ill." For abbreviations of the names of states, see 2.13; use of two-letter postal abbreviations is discouraged by some institutions. Distinguish between Cambridge, England, and Cambridge, Massachusetts. Unless otherwise indicated by the state name or the name of an institution such as Harvard University, the English city will be assumed.

8.54   For foreign cities, use the English name if there is one: Cologne, not Köln; Munich, not München; Florence, not Firenze; Padua, not Padova; Milan, not Milano; Rome, not Roma; Vienna, not Wien; Prague, not Praha; and so forth.

8.55   Follow the place of publication with a colon if a publisher is given, with a comma if only the date follows. If neither the title page nor the copyright page gives the place of publication, write *n.p.* (for *no place*) as the first fact of publication.

8.56   The abbreviation *n.p.* may also stand for *no publisher.* If both place and publisher are missing, *n.p.* with the date is sufficient.

8.57   *Name of publishing agency.* The broader term *publishing agency,* rather than *publisher,* is used here because some of the works are published by societies, institutions of learning or commerce or banking, and the like that are not publishers per se. The terms are used interchangeably in the text of this section. After place of publication and a colon followed by one space, the name of the publisher may be given either in the style used by the company itself or in the accepted abbreviated form listed for American publishers in *Books in Print,* issued annually by R. R. Bowker Company, and for British publishers in *Whitaker's Books in Print,* published by J. Whitaker & Sons and R. R. Bowker.

8.58 Note carefully the spelling and punctuation of publishers' names. There is no comma in Houghton Mifflin, for example, but there are commas in Little, Brown and in the former Harcourt, Brace. Hyphens are used in McGraw-Hill Book Company and in Appleton-Century-Crofts. There is a small *m,* not a capital, in the middle of Macmillan.

8.59 Publishers' names may be written in full, but in notes it is customary to omit an initial *The* and the abbreviations *Inc., Ltd.,* and *S.A.* The ampersand (&) may be used in place of *and,* and *Company, Brothers,* and the like may be abbreviated (*Co., Bros.*) or omitted. The word *Press* should not be dropped from the name of a university press. The name of a publisher may also be shortened, such as "Knopf" (Alfred A. Knopf, Inc.), "Norton" (W. W. Norton and Company), and "Scribner" (Charles Scribner's Sons). Whatever style is chosen, it must be used consistently throughout the paper.

8.60 If the title page indicates that a work was copublished, the reference should give both publishers:

```
(New York: Alfred A. Knopf and Viking Press, 1966)

(Boston: Ginn & Co.; Montreal: Round Press, 1964)
```

8.61 The title page of a book issued by a subsidiary of a publisher gives both names, and references to such a book should include both:

```
(Cambridge: Harvard University Press, Belknap Press,
1965)
```

8.62 If a work has been published for an institution or association whose name appears on the title page along with the publisher, the reference should include both names:

```
(New York: Columbia University Press for American
Geographical Society, 1947)
```

8.63   If a work has been reissued since the original publication, that will usually be noted in the library catalog. Such information is especially useful for locating some hard-to-find old works. See 8.46 for the style of reference used in citing a reprint edition.

8.64   Do not substitute the present name of a publishing firm for that shown on the title page.

8.65   Do not translate parts of the names of foreign publishers, even when you have anglicized the name of the city (see 8.54). Do not, for example, change *Compagnie* or *Cie* to *Company* or *Co.;* or *et Frère* to *and Brother* or *and Bro.* They often may be omitted, however.

8.66   In a long-established practice within some scientific fields, the names of publishers are routinely omitted from citations. Thus only place and date of publication appear: for example, New York, 1970. Note that when only two facts of publication are given, they are separated by a comma.

8.67   *Date of publication.* The copyright date is used in a reference unless a different date appears with the publisher's imprint on the title page or on the copyright page itself; the latter would then be the one to use. There may be more than one copyright date; if so, use the last one. There may also be one or more dates shown in addition to the date of copyright. Since those refer to reprintings, or new impressions, not to new editions, they should not be given for the date of publication. If no date is shown anyplace, write *n.d.* (*no date*):

```
(New York: Grosset and Dunlap, n.d.)
```

8.68   If, however, the date has been established by means other than the title page or copyright date, place it in brackets. The entry for the work in the card catalog often carries the date of publication when the title page omits it. When the date has been discovered through the efforts of the library, it will be shown in brackets on the catalog card. In a note, it is given thus:

```
(New York: Grosset and Dunlap, [1831])
```

8.69   If it is desirable to cite a book that has been accepted for publication but is not yet published, use the following style:

```
        ⁶Douglas F. Stotz et al., Neotropical Birds:
Ecology and Conservation, forthcoming.
```

If the book is actually being typeset or printed, use *in press:*

```
⁷Marc Shell, Art and Money (Chicago: University of
Chicago Press, in press).
```

PAGE REFERENCES

8.70 Refer to page(s) by number alone, whether in arabic or lower-case roman numerals (for preliminaries). The abbreviations *p.* and *pp.* should precede page numbers only where their absence might cause confusion. Refer to inclusive page numbers using the system in 2.67. For use of a colon before page numbers in references to multivolume works see 8.80, and in references to articles, 8.101.

8.71 The first reference to an article in a periodical may be to a specific page or pages, as with a quotation. Inclusive page numbers for the whole article need be given only when the entire article is being cited. Use exact inclusive page numbers rather than such designations as 80 f. (80 and following page) or 82, 83 ff. (82, 83, and following pages). Since *f.* refers to only a single page immediately following the number given, the exact pages can be substituted 80–81. Similarly, give inclusive pages rather than using *ff.:* 82, 83–85.

8.72 Although inclusive page numbers are desirable in referring to an article as a whole, they should not be given when an article begins in the front of a magazine and skips to the back. In this case inclusive pages are meaningless, and the first page number alone should be cited (see 11.41).

8.73 The word *passim* (*here and there*) should be used with discretion. Employ it only in referring to information scattered over a considerable stretch of text or throughout a chapter or other long section. Give the inclusive page numbers or the chapter number and place passim at the end of the reference:

```
1. Jean Comaroff, Body of Power, Spirit of
Resistance: The Culture and History of a South African
People (Chicago: University of Chicago Press, 1985),
chap. 1 passim.
```

Note that passim is a whole word and not an abbreviation and therefore is not followed by a period unless it comes at the end of a citation. Do not italicize or underline it.

MULTIVOLUME WORKS

8.74 The publication plan of a multivolume work is more or less clearly defined in advance. The work consists, or will consist, of a limited number of volumes related to the same subject. The volumes may all be the work of one author and bear the same title (note 1); or they may be by one author and have different titles (note 2); or they may be by different authors and bear different titles, with the entire work carrying an overall title and having a general editor (note 3):

> ¹Muriel St. Clare Byrne, ed., *The Lisle Letters* (Chicago: University of Chicago Press, 1981), 6:38.

> ²William Makepeace Thackeray, *The Complete Works* (Boston, 1899), vol. 13, *The English Humorists of the Eighteenth Century,* 121–330.

> ³Eric Cochrane and Julius Kirshner, eds., *The Renaissance,* vol. 5 of *University of Chicago Readings in Western Civilization,* ed. John W. Boyer and Julius Kirshner (Chicago: University of Chicago Press, 1986), 402.

8.75 A reference to a multivolume work as a whole should include the total number of volumes.

> 1. Paul Tillich, *Systematic Theology,* 3 vols. (Chicago: University of Chicago Press, 1951–63).

A reference to one of the volumes of a multivolume work may follow one of the styles discussed in paragraphs 8.78–82. See also 8.76–77.

8.76 If the individual volumes have been issued in different years, the reference to the work as a whole must indicate that fact:

> 2. John Dryden, *The Works of John Dryden,* ed. H. T. Swedenberg, 8 vols. (Berkeley and Los Angeles: University of California Press, 1956–62).

8.77 When the publication of a multivolume work is not complete, give the date when publication began followed by a hyphen:

> 1968–

8.78 The following style should be used when referring to the whole of a specific volume in a multivolume work:

> ²Paul Tillich, *Systematic Theology,* vol. 2 (Chicago: University of Chicago Press, 1957).

8.79 When all the volumes in a multivolume work were published in the same year, only one publication date is required:

³Gordon N. Ray, ed., *An Introduction to
Literature,* vol. 2, *The Nature of Drama,* by Hubert
Hefner (Boston: Houghton Mifflin Co., 1959).

8.80 When all the volumes in a multivolume work have the same title, a reference to pages within a single volume is given in the following manner:

⁵Pierre de Ronsard, *Les oeuvres de Pierre de
Ronsard: Texte de 1587,* ed. Isidore Silver (Chicago:
University of Chicago Press, 1970), 8:55.

Note that the page reference follows the volume number and that the two are separated by a colon. Note also that the volume number is given in arabic numerals, even when expressed in roman numerals in the work cited, and that the abbreviation *vol.* is omitted.

8.81 When each volume in a multivolume work has a different title, a reference to pages within a single volume is given as follows:

1. Gabriel Marcel, *The Mystery of Being,* vol. 2,
Faith and Reality (Chicago: Henry Regnery, 1960), 19-
20.

8.82 When, in addition to volume and page, another division of a work is needed to locate a reference, that division must be appropriately designated even though the abbreviations *vol.* and *p.* are omitted:

2. Donald Lach, *Asia in the Making of Europe*
(Chicago: University of Chicago Press, 1965), 2, bk.
1:165.

8.83 The use of arabic rather than roman numerals for volume numbers is noted in 8.80. Arabic numerals are also used, with a few exceptions, for all the divisions of a written work: parts, volumes, books, chapters, pages; acts and scenes of a play; lines and stanzas of a poem; columns of a tabulation; figures, tables, and maps; and so on. There are two exceptions: (1) references to a book's preliminary pages that are numbered with lower-case roman numerals should use the same style of numerals (8.70); (2) references to divisions of unpublished public documents or to manuscript materials should follow the numbering style of the source (see 8.131–32 and 2.25).

SUBSEQUENT REFERENCES

8.84 Once a work has been cited in complete form, later references to it are shortened. For this, either short titles or the Latin abbreviation *ibid.* (for *ibidem,* "in the same place") should be used. The use of *op. cit.* and *loc. cit.,* formerly common in scholarly references, is now discouraged.

IBID.

8.85   When references to the same work follow one another with no intervening references, even though they are separated by several pages, ibid. may take the place of the author's name, the title of the work, and as much of the succeeding material as is identical. The author's name and the title are never used with ibid.

>   1. Max Plowman, *An Introduction to the Study of Blake* (London: Gollancz, 1982), 32.

With no intervening reference, a second mention of the same page of Plowman's work requires only ibid. Notice that ibid. is not italicized or underlined.

>   2. Ibid.

The following reference is to a different page:

>   3. Ibid., 68.

Ibid. may also replace the name of a journal or book of essays in successive references to that same work within one note.

8.86   Ibid. must not be used for an author's name in references to two works by the same author. The author's name may be repeated, or in references *within one note* to additional works by the same author, *idem* ("the same," sometimes abbreviated *id.*) may be used. In note 2 below, ibid. stands for all the elements of the preceding reference except the page number; in note 5 idem stands for only the author.

>   [1]Arthur Waley, *The Analects of Confucius* (London: George Allen & Unwin, 1938), 33.
>
>   [2]Ibid., 37.
>
>   [3]Arthur Waley, *Chinese Poems* (London: George Allen & Unwin, 1946), 51.
>
>   [4]Ibid., 17.
>
>   [5]Ibid., 19; idem, *The Analects of Confucius*, 25.

Note that idem is a complete word, not an abbreviation, and is therefore not followed by a period.

8.87 References following legal style, however, employ idem (abbreviated id.) where this manual stipulates ibid. Legal style reserves ibid. for references where there is no change in page or other part from the preceding reference. This special application of ibid. and idem as set forth in *A Uniform System of Citation,* fifteenth edition, should be used only in the field of law.

SHORTENED REFERENCES

8.88 Reference to a work that has already been cited in full form, but not in a note immediately preceding, is made in one of two styles, here called method A and method B. Method A uses the author's family name; title of book, chapter, or article (sometimes shortened); and specific page reference. Method B uses the author's family name and a specific page reference and includes the title of the book, chapter, or article only when two or more works by the same author are cited. For examples of method A and method B, see 8.90–91.

8.89 In both methods, for multiauthor works use the family name of each author up to three, and the first author's name plus et al. for more than three. To avoid ambiguity, the author (or authors) must be given in the note whether or not the name appears close to the citation in the text.

8.90 *Method A.* The first three notes below contain first, and therefore full, references. Notes 4 and 5 show subsequent references given in the style of method A.

> ¹Max Plowman, *Introduction to the Study of Blake* (London: Gollancz, 1952), 58-59.

> ²Max Plowman, *William Blake's Design for "The Marriage of Heaven and Hell"* (London: Faber and Faber, 1960), ix-xii.

> ³Abdul al-Achmad, *Immunization and Chemotherapy* (Chicago: Blitzstein, 1994), 247.

Note 4 refers to the first-mentioned work of Plowman, given in full in note 1, and uses the short title:

> ⁴Plowman, *Study of Blake,* 125.

Note 5 gives a second, or subsequent, reference to al-Achmad's book, first cited in note 3, and uses a short title, as required by method A, even though the book is the only work by the author previously cited:

⁵Al-Achmad, *Immunization and Chemotherapy*, 381.

8.91 *Method B.* The following notes present later references to the same sources cited in full in the first three notes in 8.90. Here the subsequent references are given in the style of method B. Note 4 makes a second reference to the work by Plowman first cited in note 2. Since two works by this author have been cited, the shortened reference must contain a shortened version of the title:

⁴Plowman, *Blake's Design*, 25.

Note 5 contains a second reference to al-Achmad's book. Since only one work by this author has been previously mentioned, the name and page number are sufficient under method B:

⁵Al-Achmad, 382.

8.92 A second or subsequent reference to a multivolume work already cited in full form, but not in the reference immediately preceding, omits the subtitle, if any; facts of publication; series title, if any; edition (unless more than one edition of the same work has been cited); and total number of volumes. Note the full reference in note 1 and a later reference to the work as shown in (arbitrarily numbered) note 9 (method A) and note 10 (method B):

1. Gabriel Marcel, *The Mystery of Being* (Chicago: Henry Regnery, 1960), 1:42.

9. Marcel, *Mystery of Being,* 2:98–99.

or

10. Marcel, 2:98–99.

Now consider another multivolume work, which has an overall title and different titles for the individual volumes, only one of which is referred to in the notes:

2. Tucker Brooke, *The Renaissance (1500–1600),* vol. 2 of *A Literary History of England,* ed. Albert C. Baugh (New York: Appleton-Century-Crofts, 1948), 104.

3. Brooke, *Renaissance,* 130.

Or in the style of method B:

3. Brooke, 130.

8.93 For a subsequent reference to a chapter in a book or to an essay, poem, or the like in an anthology, omit the name of the book and also omit the volume number, if any, and the date. The reference should consist of the author's last name (methods A and B), the title of the work in shortened form (method A only), and the page number.

8.94   *Short titles.* Titles of five or fewer words need not be shortened unless the words are very long. The following title could be shortened as shown:

`The Essential Tension: Selected Studies in Scientific`
`Tradition and Change`

shortened to

`Essential Tension`

8.95   A short title uses the key words of the main title, omitting an initial article when the title is in English. For titles beginning with such words as "A Dictionary of," "Readings in," and "An Index to" one would normally omit those words, using the topic as the short title:

`A Guide to Rehabilitation of the Handicapped`

shortened to

`Rehabilitation`

or, if necessary to avoid confusion with similar titles by the same author,

`Rehabilitation of the Handicapped`

`Bibliography of North American Folklore and Folksong`

shortened to

`Folklore and Folksong`

If possible, the word order should not be changed. There are, however, dictionaries and bibliographies that cover a variety of topics: *An Index to General Literature, Biographical, Historical, and Literary Essays and Sketches, Reports and Publications of Boards and Societies Dealing with Education.* It would not do to include only one category; the only reasonable short title is simply *Education Index.*

8.96   When a short title might cause confusion, the first, full citation of the work should note that short title:

`(hereafter cited as Education Index)`

PERIODICALS

8.97   Periodicals are publications issued at regular intervals. There are three major categories: journals, magazines, and newspapers. Journals and magazines may be distinguished by their usual content and breadth of readership; journals tend to be more scholarly and more specialized and to have a more limited circulation. Citations to journals and to magazines usually differ in only one respect: whereas journal citations include volume or issue number, citations to magazines ordinarily refer to date only.

8.98   References to periodicals normally omit place and publisher (newspaper names do, however, include place; see 8.105–10), except that for foreign periodicals of limited circulation and titles that are identical or similar to those of periodicals published elsewhere, the place of publication should be added in parentheses:

> [1]Jack Fishman, "Un grand homme dans son intimité: Churchill," *Historia* (Paris), no. 220 (November 1964): 684-94.

JOURNALS

8.99   The first, full reference to an article in a periodical includes, in general, the following facts in the order shown:

> author(s)
> title of article
> title of periodical
> volume or issue number (or both)
> publication date
> page number(s)

In note citations, these information elements are separated by commas, except that dates are enclosed in parentheses and a colon introduces the page reference. As with books, however, in bibliographic entries the elements are separated by periods.

8.100   Authors' names are treated as they are in references to books (see 8.26–36). Article titles are put in quotation marks, and the titles of periodicals are italicized or underlined and capitalized headline style (both English language and foreign).

²W. Edmund Farrar, "Antibiotic Resistance in Developing Countries," *Journal of Infectious Diseases* 152 (December 1985): 1103.

8.101   Volume numbers and issue numbers are given in arabic numerals following the name of the journal. When the citation is to specific pages, no abbreviation precedes the volume number or the page numbers, but an issue number is preceded by *no.* The issue number is required only if issues are paginated separately rather than in sequence throughout the volume. The date of publication is enclosed in parentheses and follows the volume and any issue number—the month or season can generally be omitted if an issue number is given. There is no punctuation between the name of the journal and the volume number, and none between the month and year. A colon separates the date from the page reference.

1. John J. Benjoseph, "On the Anticipation of New Metaphors," *Cuyahoga Review* 24 (1988): 6-10.

2. Cartright C. Bellworthy, "Reform of Congressional Remuneration," *Political Review* 7, no. 6 (1990): 89, 93-94.

3. Jane R. Bush, "Rhetoric and the Instinct for Survival," *Political Perspectives* 29 (March 1990): 45-53.

4. Ilya Bodonski, "Caring among the Forgotten," *Journal of Social Activism* 14 (fall 1989): 112-34.

Some journals are not published in volumes but only in issues. In that case the year of publication may be said to take the place of a volume number. There are two ways of presenting such a reference:

⁵Patrick Skelton, "Rehabilitation versus Demolition," *Journal of Urban Renewal,* no. 3 (1989): 145.

or

⁵Patrick Skelton, "Rehabilitation versus Demolition," *Journal of Urban Renewal* 1989, no. 3:145.

Note that when the issue number (identified by *no.*) comes first, it follows a comma and the year is enclosed in parentheses. When the year comes first, however, serving as a volume number, it is not preceded by a comma or enclosed in parentheses. In both cases a colon precedes the page reference, but in the second instance there is no space after it.

8.102 Some periodicals publish volumes in successive series, each beginning with volume 1. In some cases the series are numbered, in some they are lettered, and in some they are designated *old series* or *new series,* abbreviated *o.s.* and *n.s.* This information must be noted in the reference. Note that the series designation is set off by commas.

> 1. "Letters of Jonathan Sewall," *Proceedings of the Massachusetts Historical Society,* 2d ser., 10 (January 1896): 414.

> 2. G. M. Moraes, "St. Francis Xavier, Apostolic Nuncio, 1542-52," *Journal of the Bombay Branch of the Royal Asiatic Society,* n.s., 26 (1950): 279-313.

8.103 The proper style for citing articles is not likely to raise questions except when an entire issue of a publication is devoted to one long paper. Sometimes such an issue replaces the usual issue, bearing its number in the succession; sometimes it bears a supplementary number. In either case the question is, Should the citation conform to the style used for a whole publication or to that used for an article? The answer lies in the view taken by the publishers of periodicals and by librarians, that a paper occupying a whole issue is published *in* the periodical. Thus it is cited as an article, except that the special designation shown on the cover of the particular issue is included in the reference (e.g., supplement, special issue):

> [1]Elias Folker, "Report on Research in the Capital Markets," *Journal of Finance* 39, suppl. (May 1964): 15.

MAGAZINES

8.104 Magazines of general interest, even though they may carry volume numbers, are best identified by date alone. The date then takes the place of the volume number and is not enclosed in parentheses, but the periodical name is followed by a comma.

> [4]Anne B. Fisher, "Ford Is Back on the Track," *Fortune,* 23 December 1985, 18.

> [2]Michael Rogers, "Software for War, or Peace: All the World's a Game," *Newsweek,* 9 December 1985, 82.

NEWSPAPERS

8.105 For reference to a newspaper, the name of the paper and the date are sufficient; but many large metropolitan papers—especially Sunday editions—are made up of sections that are separately paginated. For these, section number (or letter), page number, and edition letter (often in uppercase) must be given. It is convenient for the reader if the title of the article and the name of the author, if given, are included in the reference:

    ⁷Tyler Marshall, "200th Birthday of Grimms
Celebrated," *Los Angeles Times,* 15 March 1985, sec. 1A,
p. 3.

    ²Michael Norman, "The Once-Simple Folk Tale
Analyzed by Academe," *New York Times,* 5 March 1984,
15(N).

8.106 If the name of an American newspaper does not include the city, add the city before the newspaper title and italicize or underline both. If the city is not widely known, give the state in parentheses:

Houlton (Maine) Pioneer Times
Hiawatha (Kans.) Daily World

8.107 If the name of the city is the same as that of a better-known city, add the name of the state or province in parentheses:

Ottawa (Ill.) Times
St. Paul (Alberta) Journal

8.108 For foreign newspapers in which the city of publication is not part of the title, the city should be given in parentheses after the title:

Times (London)
Le Monde (Paris)

but

Frankfurter Zeitung
Manchester Guardian

8.109 The city of publication need not be given for such well-known newspapers as the *Christian Science Monitor,* the *Wall Street Journal,* and the *National Observer.*

8.110 An initial *the* in English language newspaper titles is omitted, but its equivalent in a foreign language is retained: thus, *Times* (London) but *Le Monde* (Paris). This practice holds for notes, bibliographies, and reference lists. When a newspaper (or journal or magazine) title appears in the text, *the* may precede the name if the syntax requires it, but it is not treated as part of the title:

The Sunday edition of the *San Francisco Examiner* includes an excellent section on entertainment.

The *New York Times* gives superior coverage to foreign news.

He prefers *New York Times* editorials to those of any other newspaper.

SUBSEQUENT REFERENCES

8.111   Subsequent references to articles, reviews, and other pieces published in periodicals may be shortened by omitting the periodical title and issue information and, if necessary, shortening the title of the piece. Only the last name of the author is used unless there are others by that name. When no author is given, the title comes first. The following are shortened versions of some of the full references in 8.98–105:

Journals

8. Fishman, "Un grand homme," 691.

9. Farrar, "Antibiotic Resistance," 1104.

10. Benjoseph, "New Metaphors," 7, 9.

11. Bellworthy, "Congressional Remuneration," 93-94.

12. "Letters of Sewall," 414.

13. Moraes, "St. Francis Xavier," 280-87.

Magazines

14. Fisher, "Ford Is Back," 18.

Newspapers

15. Marshall, "200th Birthday," sec. 1A, p. 3.

16. Norman, "Once-Simple Folk Tale," 15(N).

SPECIAL FORMS

ARTICLES IN ENCYCLOPEDIAS AND DICTIONARIES

8.112   Well-known reference books are generally not listed in bibliographies. When they are cited in notes, the facts of publication (place of publication, publisher, and date) are usually omitted, but the edition, if not the first, must be specified. In encyclopedias that are under continuous revision, however, no edition might be mentioned on the title page, and the copyright date should be included (note 2 below). References to an encyclopedia, dictionary, or other alphabetically arranged work cite the title of the entry (not the volume or page number) preceded by *s.v.* (*sub verbo,* "under the word"). For an entry that extends to several pages, however, provide the page number unless the reference is to the entire article. For a signed article, the name of the author may be included. (If only initials appear with the entry, the list of authors in the front matter may provide the name.)

¹*Encyclopaedia Britannica,* 11th ed., s.v. "Blake, William," by J. W. Cosyns-Carr.

²*Encyclopedia Americana,* 1963 ed., s.v. "Sitting Bull."

³*Columbia Encyclopedia,* 3d ed., s.v. "Cano, Juan Sebastian del."

⁴*Webster's New Geographical Dictionary* (1984), s.v. "Dominican Republic."

An alternative form is to cite the author, if known, and the name of the article first, followed by the title of the encyclopedia or dictionary and information about the edition or the date of publication:

¹J. W. Cosyns-Carr, "Blake, William," in *Encyclopaedia Britannica,* 11th ed.

NOVELS, PLAYS, AND POEMS

NOVELS

8.113   References to novels are treated exactly like references to nonfiction books. The particular edition referred to must be specified in the first reference, with a comment telling the reader if subsequent citations will be to that edition:

3. James Joyce, *Ulysses,* a critical and synoptic edition prepared by Hans Walter Gabler with Wolfhard Steppe and Claus Melchior, 3 vols. (New York: Garland, 1984), 1:177 (all subsequent references are to this edition).

A subsequent reference would be as follows:

>   9. Joyce, *Ulysses,* 2:34-35.

See also 8.84–96.

8.114   References to modern plays follow the style for books, except that act, scene, and line numbers are given instead of pages when the page number alone is not adequate. Note that *lines* is not abbreviated.

>   ¹David Mamet, *The Poet and the Rent: A Play for Kids from Seven to 8:15* (New York: French, 1981), 35.

>   ²Jean Anouilh, *Antigone,* ed. Raymond Laubreaux, Classiques de la civilisation française, ed. Yves Brunswick and Paul Givestier (Paris: Editions de la Table Ronde, 1946; Didier, 1964), lines 1678-79, p. 87.

8.115   The classical reference style described in 8.119–27 may be adapted for citations to classic English works in which sections (acts, scenes, parts, books, cantos) and lines are numbered. Punctuation may be omitted between elements as for Greek and Latin references, or it may be included.

Romeo and Juliet, 3.2.1-30

>   for

Romeo and Juliet, act 3, scene 2, lines 1-30

>   *or*

Paradise Lost 1.83-86

>   for

Paradise Lost, book 1, lines 83-86

For works of widely known authors, the author's name is frequently omitted. Among such works are the plays of Shakespeare and Jonson and such well-known long poems as *The Faerie Queene, Paradise Lost,* and *The Ring and the Book.* The title is italicized or underlined, whether the work is published as a separate volume or as part of a collection, and the facts of publication are given in the first reference but may be omitted in subsequent references. It is important to identify the edition used, since variations occur in wording, line numbering, and even scene division.

3. *Hamlet,* Arden edition, ed. Harold Jenkins (London: Methuen, 1982), 4.5.17-20.

4. *Hamlet,* Arden, 5.2.215-20.

SHORT POEMS

8.116   To cite short poems, which most often are published in collections, the title is placed in quotation marks and the name of the collection is italicized or underlined. Stanzas, lines, and pages may be included. When quoting poems in their entirety in a thesis or dissertation, it may be necessary to obtain permission (see 5.1).

REVIEWS

8.117   In a first reference to a review, give the name of the reviewer; the title of the review (if any); the phrase *review of* followed by an identification of the work reviewed, as illustrated in the examples below; and finally the book, periodical, or newspaper in which the review appears.

Book reviews:

[1]Steven Spitzer, review of *The Limits of Law Enforcement,* by Hans Zeisel, *American Journal of Sociology* 91 (November 1985): 726-29.

[2]David Scott Kastan, review of *Jonson's Gypsies Unmasked: Background and Theme of "The Gypsies Metamorphos'd,"* by Dale B. J. Randall, *Modern Philology* 76 (May 1979): 391-94.

[3]Susan Lardner, "Third Eye Open," review of *The Salt Eaters,* by Toni Cade Bambara, *New Yorker,* 5 May 1980, 169.

Play reviews:

[4]Review of *Fool for Love,* by Sam Shepard, as performed by the Circle Repertory Company, New York, *New York Times,* 27 May 1983, 18(N).

Reviews of televised plays:

[5]Review of a televised version of *True West,* by Sam Shepard, *New York Times,* 31 January 1984, 22(N).

INTERVIEWS

8.118   References to interviews include the name of the person or group interviewed; any interview title in quotation marks; the words *interview by* followed by the interviewer's name; the medium in which the interview appeared—whether a book, journal, radio or television program, or some other form—in italics or quotation marks as it would be in any reference; the name of any editor, translator, or director (8.40–42); and the facts of publication or other information required for locating printed or nonprinted sources:

> 1. Raymond Bellour, "Alternation, Segmentation, Hypnosis: Interview with Raymond Bellour," interview by Janet Bergstrom, *Camera Obscura,* nos. 3-4 (summer 1979): 93.

> 2. Isaac Bashevis Singer, interview by Harold Flender, in *Writers at Work: The "Paris Review" Interviews,* ed. George Plimpton, 5th ser. (New York: Viking Press, 1981), 85.

> 3. Horace Hunt [pseud.], interview by Ronald Schatz, tape recording, 16 May 1976, Pennsylvania Historical and Museum Commission, Harrisburg.

References to interviews conducted by the author of a paper should include the name of the person interviewed; a description of the type of interview capitalized sentence style; and the place and date of the interview:

> 4. Merle A. Roemer, interview by author, tape recording, Millington, Md., 26 July 1973.

GREEK AND LATIN CLASSICAL WORKS

8.119   References to classical works use abbreviations for the author's name; for the title of the work; for collections of inscriptions, papyri, ostraca, and so on; and for the titles of well-known periodicals and other reference tools. For a list of accepted abbreviations, consult the *Oxford Classical Dictionary* (see also 2.22). Such abbreviations should be used only in papers on predominantly classical topics, however. Sample notes appear in 8.127 below.

8.120   Titles of individual works, collections, and periodicals are italicized or underlined, whether given in full or abbreviated. In

Greek and Latin titles, only the first word, proper nouns, and proper adjectives are capitalized.

8.121 The different levels of division of a work (book, part, section, chapter, line, etc.) are given in arabic numerals. When designated by number only, the levels are separated by periods (with no spaces following):

> ¹Stat. *Silv.* 1.3.32.

References to the same level are separated by commas:

> ²Ovid *Met.* 1.240, 242.

A hyphen separates inclusive numbers (see 8.127, sample notes 1, 2, 8, 9). If, for clarity, identifying abbreviations are used before the numbers, the divisions are separated by commas, not periods (bk. 2, sec. 4).

8.122 There is no punctuation between the author's name and the title of the work, and none between the title and the first reference unless it includes an identifying word or abbreviation, which should be preceded by a comma (see 8.127, notes 3 and 4). (In papers where classical references are mixed with other references, it is acceptable to put a comma after the author's name.)

8.123 In general the facts of publication are omitted, but the name of the edition may be given after the title (8.127, note 4), and it *must be given* if the reference is to page numbers rather than to book, chapter, and so on.

8.124 The number of an edition other than the first is indicated by a superior number placed either after the title (8.127, note 8) or, if the reference includes a volume number, after that (8.127, note 7).

8.125 A superior letter or figure placed immediately after a number referring to a division of a work (other than a volume) indicates a subdivision (8.127, note 9). If preferred, the letters may be placed on the line, and either capital or small letters may be used, depending on usage in the source cited.

8.126 Arabic numerals are now generally used in references to volumes in collections of inscriptions. Periods follow the volume number and the inscription number, and further subdivisions are treated as in other classical references. Although it is not necessary, a comma may follow the title (or the abbreviation

of the title) provided the usage is consistent in similar references (see 8.127, note 6).

8.127   The following examples illustrate points discussed in 8.119–26.

> [1]Homer *Odyssey* 9.266-71.

or

> [2]Hom. *Od.* 9.266-71.

> [3]Cicero *De officiis* 1.133, 140.

> [4]Horace *Satires, Epistles and Ars Poetica,* Loeb
> Classical Library, p. 12.

> [5]H. Musurillo *TAPA* 93 (1926): 231.

> [6]*IG Rom.* 3.739.9.10, 17.

Note 6 refers to *Inscriptiones Graecae ad res Romanas perti-
nentes,* vol. 3, document 739, section 9, lines 10 and 17.

> [7]E. Meyer *Kleine Schriften* 1^2 (Halle, 1924), 382.

> [8]Stolz-Schmalz *Lat. Gram.*^{5} (rev. Leumann-Hoffmann:
> Munich, 1928), 390-91.

> [9]Aristotle *Poetica* 20.1456^2 20.34-35.

> [10]*POxy.* 1485.

Note 10 refers to *Oxyrhynchus Papyri,* document 1485.

MEDIEVAL WORKS

8.128   References to medieval works may be in the same style as that
used for Greek and Latin classical works:

> 1. Irenaeus *Against Heresies* 1.8.3.

> 2. John of the Cross *Ascent of Mount Carmel*
> (trans. E. Allison Peers in *The Complete Works of Saint
> John of the Cross* [London: Burns, Oates, and
> Washbourne, 1934-35]) 2.20.5.

> 3. *Beowulf,* lines 2401-7.

When the specific part is named, as in note 3, a comma separates title from reference.

SCRIPTURAL REFERENCES

8.129   Exact references to the Bible and the Apocrypha use abbreviations for the books both in text and in notes. Chapter and

verse, separated by either a colon or a period (be consistent), are both given in arabic numerals. Identify which version is being cited (see 2.20–21).

> ¹Ps. 103:6-14.

> ²1 Cor. 13.1-13 NEB (New English Bible).

Non-Christian sacred scriptures are referred to in the same manner.

UNPUBLISHED MATERIAL

8.130   The question of what constitutes publication is often troublesome. For the purposes of documentary style, however, we may say that publication involves the *intention of general distribution*. A work undertaken to fulfill some personal objective— for example, a thesis, dissertation, speech, lecture, letter, or internal corporate announcement—even with the idea of general *availability* but without the intention of general distribution, may be considered unpublished. Although some ambiguity arises with the recent availability of dissertations on-line from University Microfilms, a liberal interpretation of the definition still permits including such works in the category unpublished.

8.131   When a specific unpublished document is first discussed in the paper, include the pertinent facts within the text and in summary form within the note. In the note, list the author's name first or, if using a letter, list it in conjunction with a correspondent (notes 2 and 6 below). For uncertain authorship or titles, use brackets (note 2). If no authorship can be established, begin the note with the document's title, if any, in quotation marks. If the document has both an author and a title, the title in quotation marks should follow the author's name (notes 3 and 4). The description of the document should follow the title if there is one; otherwise it follows the author's name (see note 1). Capitalize the description of the document sentence style (see 4.9) in notes or abbreviate it according to guidelines set forth in 2.19. If the document is dated, that date should follow. Next give the full name of the collection the manuscript belongs to, capitalized headline style (4.6–8). The full name of the depository follows (e.g., "Beinecke Rare Book and Manuscript Library, Yale University," not "Yale University Library"), and next its location by city and, if needed, state. Last comes the page number, if any.

> 1. Thomas Jefferson, Blank pass for a ship, 1801-1809, DS by Jefferson as president, Special Collections, Joseph Regenstein Library, University of Chicago, Chicago.

> 2. Garnett Duncan, Louisville, Kentucky, to [Joel Tanner Hart, Florence, Italy], ALS, 12 June 1961, Durrett Collection, Special Collections, Joseph Regenstein Library, University of Chicago, Chicago.

> 3. Abraham Lincoln, "Gettysburg Address" [final draft], AD [photostat], 19 November 1863, Special Collections, Joseph Regenstein Library, University of Chicago, Chicago; original in Library of Congress, Washington, D.C.

> 4. Sandra Landis Gogel, "A Grammar of Old Hebrew" (Ph.D. diss., University of Chicago, 1985), 46-50.

> 5. Eulogy of Charles V in Latin, apparently written at the monastery of St. Just, Spain, [ca. 1500], Special Collections, Joseph Regenstein Library, University of Chicago, Chicago.

> 6. Hiram Johnson to John Callan O'Laughlin, 13, 16 July, 28 November 1916, O'Laughlin Papers, Roosevelt Memorial Collection, Harvard College Library, Cambridge.

8.132   References to formal speeches or to papers read at meetings should include all of the information above in addition to the meeting and the sponsoring organization (if any), the location, and the date, all spelled out, capitalized sentence style, and placed after the name of the speaker and the title of the speech or the type of speech (e.g., eulogy, sermon, lecture). The title of the speech or paper is capitalized headline style and enclosed in quotation marks. The name and location of the depository where the unpublished manuscript is located should follow information about the meeting at which the speech was delivered (or was to be delivered):

> [1]David J. Bredehoft, "Self-Esteem: A Family Affair, an Evaluation Study" (paper presented at the annual meeting of the National Council on Family Relations, Saint Paul, Minnesota, 11-15 October 1983), ERIC, ED 240461.

> [2]Thomas Foxcroft, "A Seasonal Memento for New Year's Day" (sermon preached at the Old Church lecture in Boston on 1 January 1746-47), Beinecke Rare Book and Manuscript Library, Yale University, New Haven.

LEGAL CITATIONS

8.133 Research papers on predominantly legal topics may employ the style of reference described in *A Uniform System of Citation,* fifteenth edition, a detailed guide published by the Harvard Law Review Association, or the somewhat simpler style set forth in *The University of Chicago Manual of Legal Citation.* When papers in other disciplines refer to books and periodicals in the field of law, as is frequently done in the social sciences, for example, the references to legal works should be adapted to the style of the rest of the citations.

8.134 For citing government documents, see section 8.136 and the discussion and examples in chapter 12. For reference works and style manuals relevant to government documents, see the bibliography.

8.135 Though names of legal cases are italicized or underlined in text, they are given in roman in notes, bibliographies, and reference lists:

> 1. Thompson v. Smith, 170 F. Supp. 331 (D. Conn. 1987).

The reference begins with the names of the first plaintiff and the first defendant, capitalized. Volume name (capitalized and abbreviated) and page of the law report follow. Next come the name of the court that decided the case and the year it was decided. Note that *v.* not *vs.* is used for *versus* in such references:

> 1. United States v. Dennis, 183 F.2d 201 (2d Cir. 1950).

> 2. Bridges v. California, 314 U.S. 252 (1941).

PUBLIC DOCUMENTS

8.136 For work in some fields or disciplines it may be necessary or helpful to refer to public documents, of which there are a multitude of kinds, including congressional journals, records of debates, reports of committees and special hearings, bills, resolutions, laws, public acts, treaties, statutes, executive orders and reports, and constitutions. References to such sources should include elements needed for location through standard indexes, information services, and libraries. For a comprehensive discussion of references to public documents, and for samples comparing note-bibliography and author-date styles, see chapter 12.

MICROFORM EDITIONS

8.137 Works issued commercially in microfilm, microfiche, or textfiche (printed text and microfiche illustrations issued together) are treated much like books, except that the form of publication is given at the end of the entry (if it is not part of the name of the publisher), and a sponsoring organization may be listed as well as the publisher:

> [1]Abraham Tauber, *Spelling Reform in the United States* (Ann Arbor, Mich.: University Microfilms, 1958), 50.

> [2]Charles Wilson Peale, *The Collected Papers of Charles Wilson Peale and His Family,* ed. Lillian B. Miller, National Portrait Gallery, Smithsonian Institution, Washington, D.C. (Millwood, N.Y.: Kraus-Thomson Organization, 1980), microfiche, 37.

> [3]Harold Joachim, *French Drawings and Sketchbooks of the Nineteenth Century,* Art Institute of Chicago (Chicago: University of Chicago Press, 1978), textfiche, 1:59.

8.138 Microfilm or other photographic processes used only to preserve printed material, such as newspaper files, in a library are not mentioned in a citation. The source is treated as it would be in its original published version. Such is not the case, however, with materials obtained through computer or information services.

MATERIAL OBTAINED THROUGH LOOSE-LEAF OR INFORMATION SERVICES

8.139 References to material obtained through loose-leaf services such as the Federal Tax Service and information services such as ERIC (Educational Resources Information Center) or NTIS (National Technical Information Service) are exactly like first references to the original printed material, except that the pertinent facts within an entry are followed by the name of the service, the vendor providing the service, and the accession or identifying numbers within the service (see 12.20). If the service is revised annually, the year must be included. For some loose-leaf services, paragraphs rather than pages are given:

> [1]2 P-H 1966 Fed. Tax Serv. par. 10182.

> [2]D. Beevis, "Ergonomist's Role in the Weapon System Development Process in Canada" (Downsview, Ont.: Defence and Civil Institute of Environmental Medicine, 1983), 8, NTIS, AD-A145 5713/2, microfiche.

Some material available through computer and information services is not previously published. Treat such documents like any unpublished material (see 8.131–32), giving the name of the service, the vendor providing the service, and the accession or identifying numbers within the service at the end of the entry:

> [3]Linda B. Rudolf, "The Impact of the Divorce Process on the Family," paper presented at the twenty-ninth annual meeting of the Southeastern Psychological Association, 23-26 March 1983, 12, EDRS, ED 233277, microfiche.

COMPUTER PROGRAMS

8.140 References to computer programs, packages, languages, systems, and the like, known collectively as software, should in general include the title, usually spelled out except for such commonly known programs as FORTRAN, BASIC, or COBOL; such identifying detail as version, level, release number, or date; the short name or acronym, where applicable, along with other information necessary for identification, all in parentheses; and the location and name of the person, company, or organization having the property rights to the software. The author's name may also be mentioned if it is important for identification.

> 1. FORTRAN H-extended Version [or Ver.] 2.3, IBM, White Plains, N.Y.

> 2. Borland Delphi, Borland International, Scott's Valley, Calif., 1995.

> 3. Statistical Package for the Social Sciences Level M Ver. 8 (SPSS Lev. M 8.1), SPSS, Chicago.

> 4. Microsoft Excel Ver. 5.0a, Microsoft Corporation, Redmond, Wash., 1993.

ELECTRONIC DOCUMENTS

8.141   Electronic media are of two main types: (1) physical entities such as CD-ROMs, diskettes, and magnetic tapes, and (2) on-line sources such as computer services, networks, and bulletin boards. The former are in relatively fixed form, although they may be updated periodically; the latter may be continually revised, making the precise date of access especially important. Citations of electronic documents can follow the same general form as citations of printed materials. The same basic information is needed: author and title of the particular item; name and description of the source cited, whether CD-ROM, some other physical form, or an on-line source; city of publication, if any; publisher or vendor (or both); date of publication or access (or both); and identifying numbers or pathway needed for access to the material. Citations of material previously issued in print should include the same information and use the same style as any references to books and periodicals, as well as providing the additional information necessary to locate the electronic version.

[1]Richard D. Lanham, *The Electronic Word: Democracy, Technology, and the Arts* [diskette] (Chicago: University of Chicago Press, 1993).

[2]Robin Toner, "Senate Approves Welfare Plan That Would End Aid Guarantee," *New York Times,* 20 September 1995, national ed., A1, *New York Times Ondisc* [CD-ROM], UMI-Proquest, December 1995.

[3]Jeffrey Michael Jones, "A Survey of the Use of Household Appliances in Middle-Class American Homes, 1925-1960" (Ph.D. diss., University of Chicago, 1995), abstract in *Dissertation Abstracts International* 55 (1995): 3578A, *Dissertation Abstracts Ondisc* [CD-ROM], November 1995.

[4]*Oxford English Dictionary,* 2d ed., s.v. "glossolalia" [CD-ROM] (Oxford: Oxford University Press, 1992).

[5]Geoffery Chaucer, *The Canterbury Tales, English Poetry Full-Text Database,* rel. 2 [CD-ROM] (Cambridge: Chadwyck, 1993).

[6]Bureau of the Census, *Median Gross Rent by Counties of the United States, 1990,* prepared by the Geography Division in cooperation with the Housing Division, Bureau of the Census [CD-ROM] (Washington, D.C., 1995).

[7]United States v. Shabani, document no. 93-981. (U.S. Supreme Ct. 1994), reproduced in *SIRS Government Reporter CD-ROM* [CD-ROM] (Boca Raton, Fla.: Social Issues Resources Series, 1995).

[8]"Acquired Immunodeficiency Syndrome," in *MESH Vocabulary File* [database on-line] (Bethesda, Md.: National Library of Medicine, 1990, accessed 3 October 1990), identifier no. D000163, 49 lines.

[9]*Belle de jour,* in *Magill's Survey of the Cinema* [database on-line] (Pasadena, Calif.: Salem Press, ca. 1989-, accessed 1 January 1990); available from DIALOG Information Services, Palo Alto, Calif., accession no. 50053, p. 2 of 4.

[10]William J. Mitchell, *City of Bits: Space, Place, and the Infobahn* [book on-line] (Cambridge, Mass.: MIT Press, 1995, accessed 29 September 1995); available from http://www-mitpress.mit.edu:80/City_of_Bits/ Pulling_Glass/index.html; Internet.

[11]Joanne C. Baker and Richard W. Hunstead, "Revealing the Effects of Orientation in Composite Quasar Spectra," *Astrophysical Journal* 452:L95-L98, 20 October 1995 [journal on-line]; available from http:// ww.aas.org/ApJ/v452n2/5309/5309.html; Internet; accessed 29 September 1995.

In sample notes 10 and 11 the access path is noted in the universal resource locator (URL) format that has recently come into common use. Although the URL is a complete specification of the retrieval method for a document, it should never be substituted for the name of the publication and the publisher. Electronic journals, for example, may move to other locations on the Internet or may cease to exist as Internet publications, so a citation giving only the URL becomes meaningless. In time the infrastructure may permit more abstract methods of accessing materials on the Internet; a scheme using universal resource names (URN) is being planned, providing a canonical name, not specific to a machine, that applies even when a document is moved to another location. We recommend using such abstract retrieval schemes as they become available.

MUSICAL SCORES

8.142 References to published musical scores follow rules similar to those for books:

1. Giuseppe Verdi, *Rigoletto: Melodrama in Three Acts by Francesco Maria Piave,* ed. Martin Chusid, in *The Works of Giuseppe Verdi,* ser. 1, *Operas* (Chicago: University of Chicago Press; Milan: G. Ricordi, 1982).

2. Wolfgang Amadeus Mozart, *Sonatas and Fantasies for the Piano,* prepared from the autographs and earliest printed sources by Nathan Broder, rev. ed. (Bryn Mawr, Pa.: Theodore Presser, 1960), 42.

MUSICAL COMPOSITIONS

8.143   In references to musical compositions, first list the composer's name, then the title of the work, italicized or underlined and capitalized headline style (see 4.6–8). An instrumental composition identified only by form, number, and key should not be italicized or put in quotation marks. A published score with such a title, however, is treated like a book and italicized:

[1]Francis Poulenc, *Gloria.*

[2]Ludwig van Beethoven, Symphony no. 5 in C Minor.

[3]Charles Gounod, *Faust,* libretto by J. Barbier and M. Carré (New York: G. Schirmer, 1930), 113.

SOUND RECORDINGS

8.144   Records, tapes, compact discs, and other forms of recorded sound are generally listed under the name of the composer, writer, or other person(s) responsible for the content. Collections or anonymous works are listed by title. The title of a recording or album is italicized or underlined. If included, the name of the performer follows the title. The recording company and the number of the recording are usually sufficient identification, but the date of copyright, kind of recording (stereo, quadraphonic, four-track cassette, etc.), the number of records in an album, and so on may be added. This information may be found on the label of the recording or on its container (sleeve, box, etc.) or in printed material accompanying it. If the fact that it is a recording is not implicit in the designation from the label, a description may be added to the listing. In notes it is sometimes necessary to identify audio recordings, since disks, cassettes, and tapes may be used for video as well as sound recordings and for computer programs.

1. Johann Sebastian Bach, *The Brandenburg Concertos,* Paillard Chamber Orchestra, RCA CRL2-5801.

2. Peg Leg Howell, "Blood Red River," *The Legendary Peg Leg Howell,* Testament T-2204.

3. Archie Green, Introduction to brochure notes for Glenn Ohrlin, *The Hell-Bound Train,* University of Illinois Campus Folksong Club CFC 301, reissued as Puritan 5009.

4. *Genesis of a Novel: A Documentary on the Writing Regimen of Georges Simenon* (Tucson, Ariz.: Motivational Programming Corp., 1969), sound cassette.

5. M. J. E. Senn, *Masters and Pupils,* audiotapes of lectures by Lawrence S. Kubie, Jane Loevinger, and M. J. E. Senn, presented at meeting of the Society for Research in Child Development, Philadelphia, March 1973 (Chicago: University of Chicago Press, 1974).

VIDEORECORDINGS

8.145 References to the many varieties of audiovisual materials now available follow basically the same format. Give name of producer, director, and so forth first whenever relevant; otherwise first list the title, capitalized headline style and italicized or underlined. Next should follow any information pertinent to the purpose of the entry (e.g., cast members in a film) and the facts needed to find the source.

[1]Louis J. Mihalyi, *Landscapes of Zambia, Central Africa* (Santa Barbara, Calif.: Visual Education, 1975), slides.

[2]*The Greek and Roman World* (Chicago: Society for Visual Education, 1977), filmstrip.

[3]*An Incident in Tiananmen Square,* 16 mm, 25 min., (San Francisco: Gate of Heaven Films, 1990).

[4]L. K. Wolff, prod., *Rock-a-Bye Baby* (New York: Time-Life Films, 1971).

[5]Jean-Paul Sartre, *Sartre,* full text from a film produced by Alexandre Astruc and Michel Contat with the participation of Simone de Beauvoir, Jacques-Laurent Bost, André Gortz, and Jean Pouillon (Paris: Gallimard, 1977).

PERFORMANCES

8.146 References to performances begin with the most relevant name, whether that of the author, director, conductor, performer, or whatever. Next comes the title of the performance, in italics, though in studies of a certain play, opera, or operetta the name of the composition might come before any personal names. See 8.143 for treatment of musical compositions. Give the name of the theater and the city where the performance took place, with the name of the state (abbreviated) if needed. The date of the performance is given last.

> 1. Georg Solti, conductor, *Brandenburg Concerto no. 1* by Bach, BWV 1046, Chicago Symphony Orchestra concert, Chicago, 2 June 1985.

> 2. Placido Domingo as Don José, in *Carmen,* by Bizet, New York Metropolitan Opera, New York, 13 March 1987.

> 3. Anton Chekhov, *The Sea Gull,* Court Theatre, Chicago, 5 November 1981.

> 4. Orson Welles and the Mercury Theatre, "Invasion from Mars," radio performance, CBS, 30 October 1938, 8:00-9:00 P.M.

> 5. *Sesame Street,* television performance, PBS, 22 November 1994.

WORKS OF ART

8.147 Works of art reproduced in a book are given in the style of book references. When referring to a work of art not found as an illustration in a published source, give the artist's name first, then the title of the work of art, in italics or underlined, followed by the medium and the support (e.g., "oil on canvas"), the date, the name of the institution holding the work of art, and the location of the institution (the city and, if needed, the state or country). If the location of a work of art is unknown, use the phrase "whereabouts unknown" in parentheses. If a work of art is in a private collection and the holder prefers that its location not be given, use "private collection."

> [1]Pablo Picasso, *Crouching Woman,* oil drawing on plywood, 1946, Musée Picasso, Antibes.

> [2]Lorado Taft, *Fountain of Time,* steel-reinforced hollow-cast concrete, 1922, Washington Park, west end of Midway Plaisance, Chicago.

> [3]Lake Price, *An Interior,* print of collodon negative from 1855-56 Photographic Exchange Club album,

```
ca. 1855, International Museum of Photography at George
Eastman House, Rochester.
```

CITATIONS TAKEN FROM SECONDARY SOURCES

8.148   References to the work of one author as quoted in that of another must cite both works:

```
    1. Louis Zukofsky, "Sincerity and
Objectification," Poetry 37 (February 1931): 269,
quoted in Bonnie Costello, Marianne Moore: Imaginary
Possessions (Cambridge: Harvard University Press,
1981), 78.
```

If the purpose of such a reference is to emphasize the secondary author's quoting of the original work, use the following style:

```
    2. Bonnie Costello, Marianne Moore: Imaginary
Possessions (Cambridge: Harvard University Press,
1981), 78, quoting Louis Zukofsky, "Sincerity and
Objectification," Poetry 37 (February 1931): 269.
```

CONTENT NOTES

8.149   Content (or substantive) notes explain or amplify the textual discussion and therefore resemble the text more closely than reference notes. The source of material included in a content note may be given in one of several ways. It may be worked into a sentence, as sources are sometimes worked into the text (see notes 1 and 2 below), or it may follow as a separate item (note 3). Whether the title is cited in full and whether the facts of publication are given depend on whether the source has been referred to in a previous note:

```
    [1]Detailed evidence of the great increase in the
array of goods and services bought as income increases
is shown in S. J. Prais and H. S. Houthaker, The
Analysis of Family Budgets (Cambridge: Cambridge
University Press, 1955), table 5, 52.
```

```
    [2]Ernst Cassirer takes important notice of this in
Language and Myth (59-62) and offers a searching
analysis of man's regard for things on which his power
of inspirited action may crucially depend.
```

Since the work referred to in note 2 has already been cited in full form, only a page reference is required here.

```
        ³In 1962 the premium income received by all
voluntary health insurance organizations in the United
States was $6.3 billion, while the benefits paid out
were $7.1 billion. Health Insurance Institute, Source
Book of Health Insurance Data (New York: Health
Insurance Institute, 1963), 36, 46.
```

CROSS-REFERENCES

8.150 Occasionally a writer finds it necessary to refer to material in another part of the paper. Such references often consist simply of page or note numbers, or both, in parentheses in the text. Cross-references may also appear in notes. Whether in notes or text, however, cross-references with page numbers pose a difficulty because they can be added only after all pagination is final.

8.151 The words *above* (earlier in the paper) and *below* (later in the paper) are frequently used with cross-references because they make it clear that the reference is to the paper in hand, not to another source mentioned. *Supra* and *infra* are sometimes used, chiefly in law references, in place of above and below. See 13.17 and 13.19 for discussions of the use of computer systems to prepare papers with numbered sections that may be cross-referenced.

8.152 The word *see* is often used in cross-references; *cf.* should be used only in the sense of "compare" and is not an alternative to see. See is italicized in reference lists (10.22) but not in notes; cf. is never italicized.

```
        ¹For a detailed discussion of this matter see pp.
31-35 below.
```

8.153 A cross-reference such as "See note 3 above" intended simply to refer to the title of a source is not permissible. The regular style for subsequent references (whether following method A or method B) should be used consistently throughout the paper (see 8.84–96).

9 Bibliographies

Heading 9.2
Classification 9.3
Bibliography Entries Compared with Notes 9.7
Alphabetizing Authors' Names 9.14
Works by the Same Author 9.27
Foreign Language Titles 9.35
Annotated Bibliographies 9.36

9.1 The rules for bibliographical style in this chapter and the examples of bibliographical entries in chapter 11 apply mainly to papers in nonscientific fields, especially in the humanities. The style for reference lists in papers using parenthetical references is explained in chapter 10. Samples 14.41–42 show the correct layout on the page for a bibliography.

HEADING

9.2 The bibliography lists the sources used in writing the paper. Since a bibliography rarely includes everything that has been written on a given topic, a more accurate heading might be, for example, Selected Bibliography, Works Cited, or Sources Consulted. The last is especially suitable if the list includes such sources as personal interviews, lectures, tape recordings, radio or television broadcasts, or information available through computer services, which for convenience are commonly included.

CLASSIFICATION

9.3   The simplest, most accessible, and most broadly useful type of bibliography is a single alphabetical list. If dividing sources into various categories seems more appropriate to the work, however, a classified bibliographical style may be used. For example, in a paper using manuscript sources as well as printed works, the two kinds of sources may be put in separate sections, with manuscripts arranged either by depository or by name of collection. In a work with many references to newspapers, the newspapers may be separated from the rest of the items and listed together, each with its run of relevant dates (see 11.45). In a long bibliography listing many printed sources, books are sometimes separated from articles. In a study of the work of one person, it is usually best to list works *by* that person separately from works *about* him or her. A list of works by one author may be arranged in chronological order (by date of publication) rather than in alphabetical order. In a paper about one person, such a list may constitute the entire bibliography. Whatever the arrangement of a bibliography, no source should be listed more than once. When a bibliography is divided, a headnote sometimes lists the sections.

9.4   The topic of the paper, its thesis, and the order of presentation will determine how the bibliography should be divided. Do not, however, classify a long bibliography by themes or concepts such as love, hate, war, peace.

9.5   Sometimes the variety of source materials calls for further subdivision of the main classes under second-level subheads. For example, a section titled Primary Sources may be divided into Published Works and Unpublished Works.

9.6   Within the divisions and subdivisions, the entries should be arranged in a definite order. Although alphabetical order by family names of authors is the most common, for some papers another order—for example, chronological—is more helpful. If a scheme other than alphabetical is used, it should be explained in a headnote or in a footnote on the first page of the bibliography.

BIBLIOGRAPHY ENTRIES
COMPARED WITH NOTES

9.7   A bibliography entry includes much the same material as a
first, full note reference, arranged in the same general order.
Differences in the way of presenting this material stem from
differences in purpose. A bibliography entry is meant to identify a work in full bibliographical detail: name(s) of author(s),
full title, and place, publisher, and date of publication. The
primary purpose of a note is to inform the reader of the particular location—page, section, or other segment—from which
the writer of the paper has taken certain material cited in the
text. The secondary purpose of the note—to enable the reader
to find the source—dictates the inclusion of full bibliographical details in the first reference to a work (see 8.3). The differences in format between notes and bibliography are described
below (9.8–13) and illustrated by parallel examples in chapters
11 and 12.

9.8   The bibliography of a paper is single-spaced with one blank
line between entries. The first line of each entry is flush left,
and any runover lines are indented five spaces (see 14.41–42).

9.9   In a note the author's full name is in the natural order, given
name first, because there is no reason to invert the order. In
the bibliographical entry the family name comes first because
bibliographies are usually arranged in alphabetical order by
family names of authors:

```
McDougall, Walter A. . . . The Heavens and the Earth: A
     Political History of the Space Age. New York:
     Basic Books, 1985.
```

9.10   Where there are two or more authors' names, only the first is
inverted in the bibliography, in order to alphabetize the item.
The names following are in normal order, given name or initials first and family name last:

```
Stockwell, R. P., P. Schachter, and B. H. Partee. The
     Major Syntactic Structures of English. New York:
     Holt, Rinehart and Winston, 1973.
```

9.11   Whereas commas and parentheses separate the elements in a
note, in a bibliography entry periods are used at the end of
each main part: author's name, title of work, and facts of publication. (A single space should be left after each period.) Bibliographical references to periodicals, however, do use parenthe-

167

ses around dates of publication following volume numbers (see 11.39–40).

9.12 Page numbers are listed in bibliography entries only when the item is part of a whole work—a chapter in a book or an article in a periodical. When given, page numbers must be inclusive—first and last pages of the relevant section (see 11.40). When an article is continued at the back of a journal or magazine, however, only its first page should be given (see 8.72, 11.41).

9.13 If the institution or discipline the paper is written for requires a notation of the total number of pages for each book and pamphlet, the information is given at the end of the entry: "xiv + 450 pp."

ALPHABETIZING AUTHORS' NAMES

9.14 Bibliographies are arranged alphabetically by authors' family names, letter by letter (ignoring word spaces); in the case of identical family names, alphabetize next by given name.

9.15 Family names containing particles vary widely both in capitalization and in order of alphabetizing in bibliographies, reference lists, and indexes. The preference of the bearer—or tradition—as reflected in the biographical list at the end of *Merriam-Webster's Collegiate Dictionary* or in *Webster's New Biographical Dictionary* should be followed when alphabetizing family names with particles. Lists should be arranged letter by letter regardless of upper- and lowercase letters and intervening spaces. Such common abbreviations as *Mc* and *M* for *Mac* and *St.* and *Ste* for *Saint* and *Sainte* are alphabetized as they appear when abbreviated rather than as if they were spelled out:

```
Augustine, Saint
Becket, Saint Thomas (or Thomas à Becket, Saint
    alphabetized under the Ts)
Braun, Wernher von
D'Annunzio, Gabriele
de Gaulle, Charles
de Kooning, Willem
De La Rey, Jacobus Hercules
Della Robbia, Luca
De Mille, Agnes George
```

```
De Valera, Eamon
Deventer, Jacob Louis van
De Vere, Aubrey Thomas
De Vries, Hugo
DiMaggio, Joseph Paul
Gogh, Vincent van
Guardia, Ricardo Adolfo de la
Hindenburg, Paul von
Lafontaine, Henri-Marie
La Fontaine, Jean de
La Guardia, Fiorello Henry
Linde, Otto zur
Mabie, Hamilton Wright
Macalister, Donald
MacArthur, Douglas
Macaulay, Emilie Rose
MacMillan, Donald Baxter
Macmillan, Harold
McAdoo, William Gibbs
McAllister, Alister
M'Carthy, Justin
McAuley, Catherine Elizabeth
Ramée, Marie Louise de la
Sainte-Beuve, Charles-Augustin
Saint-Gaudens, Augustus
Saint-Saëns, Camille
St. Denis, Ruth
St. Laurent, Louis Stephen
Thomas à Kempis
Van Devanter, Willis
Van Rensselaer, Stephen
```

(handwritten: thy, Sarah — McCarthy, Sarah)

9.16   In an alternative system of alphabetizing, names beginning with abbreviated forms such as *Mc* or *M* for *Mac* and *St.* for *Saint* would be alphabetized letter by letter according to the spelled-out form even when spelled with the abbreviation. For examples, see *The Chicago Manual of Style,* fourteenth edition, 17.107 and 17.109.

9.17   Compound family names are alphabetized by the first part of the compound. For hyphenation and inversion, follow the preferences of their bearers or established usage:

```
Ap Ellis, Augustine
Campbell-Bannerman, Henry
Castelnuovo-Tedesco, Mario
Fénelon, François de Salignac de La Mothe-
```

```
Gatti-Casazza, Giulio
Ippolitov-Ivanov, Mikhail Michaylovich
La Révellière-Lépeaux, Louis-Marie de
Lloyd George, David
Mendes, Frederic de Sola
Mendès-France, Pierre
Merle d'Aubigné, Jean-Henri
Merry del Val, Rafael
Pinto, Fernão Mendes
Teilhard de Chardin, Pierre
Vaughan Williams, Ralph
Watts-Dunton, Walter Theodore
Wilson Lang, John
```

9.18   Spanish names that consist of given name (or names) and paternal and maternal family names joined with the conjunction *y* are alphabetized under the paternal name. Many names omit the conjunction, however, and in such a name as *Manuel Ramón Albeniz,* it is not clear whether the father's family name is *Ramón* or whether *Ramón* is a second given name. If the facts cannot be determined, the library catalog may serve as a guide.

9.19   Arabic, Chinese, and Japanese names should be alphabetized with particular care. In Arabic, family names beginning with *abd, abu-,* or *ibn* are usually alphabetized under these elements. Those beginning with *al-* ("the") are alphabetized by the element following this particle. The particle itself may be placed after the whole inverted name (Hakim, Tawfiq al-) or retained before it (al-Hakim, Tawfiq), which is the modern practice. Elided forms of the article (e.g., *ad-, an-, ar-*) are treated the same way, though using the elided form is discouraged by most Orientalists.

```
Hmisi, Ahmad Hamid
Husayn, Taha
al-Jamal, Muhammad Hamid
```

   or

```
Jamal, Muhammad Hamid al-
```

9.20   Chinese names usually consist of three syllables, the one-syllable family name coming first and the two-syllable given name following. In romanized form both names are capitalized: in the Wade-Giles system, the given name is hyphenated; and in pinyin, it is closed up:

PINYIN	WADE-GILES
Cheng Shifa	Ch'eng Shih-fa
Li Keran	Li K'o-jan
Zeng Youhe	Tseng Yu-ho
Zhoa Wuji	Chao Wu-chi

When alphabetizing Chinese names that are written in traditional form, even those of two instead of three syllables, the family name precedes the given name, so the name is not inverted in a bibliography or reference list, and no commas are used.

9.21 Japanese names normally consist of two elements, a family name and a given name—in that order. If the name is westernized, as it often is by authors writing in English, the order is reversed. In recent years, however, there has been a tendency among authors writing in English on Japanese subjects to use the traditional order for personal names. When alphabetizing Japanese names in a bibliography, decide how to list each entry case by case, depending on the preference of the author. Although the sequence of entries will be the same in both cases, a comma is needed with Western order:

JAPANESE ORDER	WESTERN ORDER
Kurosawa Noriaki	Kurosawa, Noriaki
Tojo Hideki	Tojo, Hideki
Yoshida Shigeru	Yoshida, Shigeru

9.22 For treatment of Hungarian names and such other non-Western names as Vietnamese, Thai, Indian, Burmese, Javanese, and Indonesian, see *The Chicago Manual of Style,* fourteenth edition, 17.113–26.

9.23 Authors with the same family name and the same first initial, when one is identified by initials alone, one by a single given name, and one by the same name plus a middle name (or initial), are alphabetized as follows:

```
Adams, J. B.
Adams, John
Adams, John Q.
Adams, John Quincy
```

9.24 When inverted, names with *Sr.* or *Jr.* or a roman numeral are punctuated as follows and arranged letter by letter:

```
Brownell, Arthur P., Jr.
Brownell, Arthur P., Sr.
```

```
Brownell, Arthur P., III
Brownell, Arthur Patrick, Jr.
```

9.25   A writer who has adopted a religious name sometimes writes under that name alone, preceded by the appropriate title. Sometimes the family name is added to the religious name. Alphabetize the name rather than the title:

```
Thérèse, Sister
Hayden, Father Cuthbert
```

9.26   Works published under a pseudonym should be listed under the pseudonym. The author's real name may be enclosed in brackets following the pseudonym if desired, and the bibliography or reference list may include a cross-reference (see 11.2 and 11.9):

```
Stendahl [Marie-Henri Beyle]          Carroll, Jenny [Meg Cabot]
Bell, Currer [Charlotte Brontë]
```

WORKS BY THE SAME AUTHOR

9.27   In a succession of works by the same author, the name is given for the first entry, and an eight-space line (the underscore key struck eight times) followed by a period takes its place in subsequent entries. The entries may be arranged alphabetically by title or chronologically. When alphabetizing titles, disregard introductory articles.

```
Eliot, T. S. Murder in the Cathedral. New York:
     Harcourt, Brace, 1935.

_____. The Sacred Wood: Essays on Poetry and
     Criticism. London: Methuen, 1920.

_____. The Waste Land. New York: Boni and
     Liveright, 1922.

     or

Eliot, T. S. The Sacred Wood: Essays on Poetry and
     Criticism. London: Methuen, 1920.

_____. The Waste Land. New York: Boni and
     Liveright, 1922.

_____. Murder in the Cathedral. New York: Harcourt,
     Brace, 1935.
```

9.28   Works edited by the author or written in collaboration with others should not be interspersed with works by the author alone. In a list including all three categories, put the edited titles after the works written by the author in question, using an eight-space line of underscores for the author's name, followed by a comma, a space, and *ed.* Translations follow (*trans.*) and then compilations (*comp.*).

9.29 Coauthored works follow edited, translated, and compiled works, but the author's name must be repeated. Do not use a line to take the place of any coauthor's name. The eight-space line of underscores may be used in place of all the names for subsequent works by the same combination of authors, however.

9.30 A long bibliography of works by one author may carry a heading including the author's name, which would then *not* appear with each item. Works edited by the author would either be listed under a subheading or begin with the abbreviation *Ed.* Works written in collaboration with others would begin, for example, "With Joseph P. Jones and John Q. Adams."

9.31 A work for which no author (editor, compiler, or other) is known appears in a bibliography under the title of the work, alphabetized by the first word, or by the first word following an initial article.

9.32 When the names of a person, a place, and a thing are spelled the same way and come at the beginning of bibliography entries, they are arranged in normal alphabetical order according to the next words in the entries.

9.33 Titles of works are capitalized and italicized or put in quotation marks according to the same rules used for notes (see 4.5–27, 8.37–39).

9.34 In some scientific fields it is customary not to italicize or underline the titles of whole publications—books, periodicals, and other works that would appear in italics in notes or text—but the same style must be followed throughout the bibliography. Quotation marks must still be used around titles of articles and other component parts of whole publications, however, as discussed in 4.15 and 4.17.

FOREIGN LANGUAGE TITLES

9.35 Use italics or quotation marks for foreign language titles just as for English titles. If an English title contains a foreign word, phrase, or title, however, it should be italicized unless the entire title is already in italics. In that case put any foreign words in quotation marks (11.21–23). Foreign language titles are generally capitalized sentence style according to the conventions of the language in question. Foreign titles contained within English titles are capitalized like English titles.

Histoire critique de l'hystérie

La litteratura italiana: Storia e testi

Aspects autobiographique de "Moby Dick" de Melville

"In Search of Gemütlichkeit"

Satires, Epistles, and Ars Poetica

ANNOTATED BIBLIOGRAPHIES

9.36   A bibliography may be annotated either in whole or in part. The annotation need not be a grammatically complete sentence, but it should begin with a capital and end with a period. The annotation begins on the line following the entry proper and should be indented at least five spaces.

Thompson, Oscar, ed. *International Cyclopaedia of Music and Musicians*. New York: Dodd, Mead, 1936.

   An admirable work that brings Grove up to date and deals adequately with contemporary music and American composers.

10 Parenthetical References and Reference Lists

Parenthetical References in the Author-Date System 10.2
Author-Date System with Notes 10.19
Reference List Style 10.20
    Cross-References 10.22
    Arrangement of Elements 10.23
Parenthetical References Using Numbers 10.33

10.1 The style of parenthetical references and reference lists recommended in *The Chicago Manual of Style,* fourteenth edition, is discussed in this chapter, and examples based on this method of citation are included in chapters 11, 12, and 14. For rules governing the use of notes and bibliographies, see chapters 8 and 9, and for examples in that style, see chapters 11, 12, and 14.

PARENTHETICAL REFERENCES IN THE AUTHOR-DATE SYSTEM

10.2 In the parenthetical, or author-date, reference system recommended in this manual, citations in running text consist of two basic elements—authors' names and dates of publication—usually in parentheses. The full biographical details for these cited works are given in a list of references arranged alphabetically by authors' family names (see 9.14–32) and chronologically within groups of works by the same author or set of authors. To aid location of a specific work, publication dates immediately follow the authors' names. The list is put at the end of the paper and may bear the title References, Works

Cited, Literature Cited, or some variation as seems appropriate.

10.3 *Author* as used here means the name under which the work is alphabetized in the reference list and may thus refer to an editor, compiler, translator, organization, or group of authors. The abbreviations *ed., comp.,* and the like are not included in the text citations but do appear in the reference list entries. There is no comma between author and date:

```
(Buttlar 1981)      (Clarke 1985)
```

If there is no date for the work, use *n.d.* (see 8.67).

```
(Lyons n.d.)
```

10.4 For works with two or three authors, give all the names (use *and,* not an ampersand):

```
(Haines and Rupp 1987)

(Wynken, Blynken, and Nodd 1988)
```

10.5 In a text reference to a work by two authors with the same last name, the family name is repeated:

```
(Weinberg and Weinberg 1980)
```

10.6 For works having more than three authors, use the name of the first followed by *et al.* or *and others.* Thus, for a work by Zipursky, Hull, White, and Israels, the parenthetical reference would read:

```
(Zipursky et al. 1995)
```

10.7 If, as sometimes happens, there is another work of the same date that would also abbreviate to "Zipursky et al."—say a paper by Zipursky, Smith, Jones, and Brown—either give the group of names in full for both or include a short title in each, set off by commas:

```
(Zipursky, Smith, Jones, and Brown 1995)
(Zipursky, Hull, White, and Israels 1995)
```

> *or*

```
(Zipursky et al., Brief notes, 1995)
(Zipursky et al., Preliminary findings, 1995)
```

10.8 Another way to distinguish such works is to cite the first two names followed by *et al.:*

```
(Zipursky, Smith, et al. 1995)
(Zipursky, Hull, et al. 1995)
```

10.9   When a book or pamphlet carries no individual author's name on the title page and is published or sponsored by a corporation, government agency, association, or other group, the name of that group may serve as the author in text references and in the reference list. Most of these names present no problem and may be used in full:

```
(International Rice Research Institute 1992)
(Federal Reserve Bank of Boston 1990)
```

10.10   For long or complex group names, text citations should be shortened. Be careful to make the citation begin with the first element of the reference list entry. For example:

```
(Ohio State University, College of Administrative
Science, Center for Human Resource Research 1993)
```

should be shortened to

```
(Ohio State University 1993)
```

rather than

```
(Center for Human Resource Research 1993)
```

Alternatively, the latter form could be used and a cross-reference added to the reference list (see also 10.22, 11.2, and 12.1):

```
Center for Human Resource Research. 1993. See Ohio
    State University. 1993.
```

10.11   Additional works by the same author cited within the same text reference are given by date only, with the dates separated by commas. If two or more of the works by a single author or set of authors have the same publication date, they are assigned the letters *a, b, c,* and so on, following the order of the reference list (see also 10.21). The letters are not italicized:

```
(García 1942, 1944)
(Keller 1896a, 1896b, 1907)
```

   or

```
(Keller 1896a,b, 1907)
```

10.12   When page numbers are given for multiple works by the same author, however, the references are separated by semicolons, and the name is repeated:

```
(Keller 1896a, 10; Keller 1896b, 4; Keller 1907, 3)
```

10.13   A specific page, section, figure, equation, or other division or element of the cited work follows the date, preceded by a comma. Unless confusion would result, *p.* or *pp.* is omitted:

```
(Rollings 1995, 15, 43)      (King 1987, eq. 57)
(Farley 1987, fig. 5)        (Black 1994, sec. 24.5)
```

10.14 When the reference is to both volume and page, a colon comes between the two. A reference to a volume only, without page number, often requires *vol.* for clarity:

```
(Kusnierek 1992, 3:125)
(García 1995, vol. 2)
(García 1995, 2:26, 35; 3:50-53)
```

10.15 Citation of a source not in the reference list, such as a personal letter or an interview, should give the full name of the letter writer or the person interviewed (unless it appears nearby in the text) and the description and date of the communication:

Spieth has indicated that some men they studied who had taken hypertensive drugs were indeed faster in psychomotor speed than nontreated hypertensives (Walter Spieth, letter to the author, June 1992).

Zebadiah Zulch (telephone interview, 1 April 1993) has maintained that he never agreed with Zipursky in the matter.

10.16 Citations to collections of unpublished manuscripts or archives may be handled by mentioning the specific item and its date, if any, in the text itself and including the collection and its depository in the reference list:

Mary E. Carpenter, a farmer's wife who lived near Rochester in 1871, listed what she did in one day at harvesting time: "My hand is so tired perhaps you'll excuse pencilling," she began a letter to her cousin Laura on 18 August.

One might add "(Carpenter Papers)" at the end of the passage above, but it is unnecessary if the name mentioned in the text is the same as the name of the collection in the reference list, so that there could be no confusion with another collection. The reference list entry would read:

Carpenter, Mary E. Lovell, and Family Papers, Minnesota Historical Society, St. Paul.

10.17 For more examples of unpublished materials in parenthetical references and reference lists, see 11.52–56.

10.18 A parenthetical reference should be placed just before a mark of punctuation:

```
Before discussing our methods of analysis, it is
necessary to describe the system of scaling
quantitative scores (Guilford 1950).
```

If this placement is impractical, the reference should be inserted at a logical place in the sentence:

```
One investigator (Carter 1990) has reported findings at
variance with the foregoing.
```

Note that if the author's name is part of the sentence, only the date is enclosed in parentheses:

```
It is true, however, that Carter (1990) has reported
findings at variance with the foregoing.
```

AUTHOR-DATE SYSTEM WITH NOTES

10.19 Sometimes a content note (see 8.149) or an acknowledgment of permission granted may be called for in a paper using parenthetical references. Such notes may appear as footnotes or endnotes (be consistent), based on the specific requirements of a particular paper, though it is usually better to include such information in the text.

```
    1. This notion seems to have something in common
with Piaget's (1977) concept of nonbalance and
equilibrium in the area of knowledge.
```

Or in text, use the following style:

```
Jones's theory, which seems to have something in common
with Piaget's (1977) concept of nonbalance and
equilibrium in knowledge, was actually developed at the
local clinic.
```

REFERENCE LIST STYLE

10.20 When the author-date system is used, references should be arranged in one alphabetical list (see sample 14.39), following the guidelines in 9.14–32.

10.21 When several works by the same author or group of authors are cited, authors' names in the reference list may stand alone, on a separate line, with their works listed below by year (see sample 14.40). As illustrated in the same sample, several works by the same author or group of authors that are published in the same year are alphabetized by title, and the publication dates are assigned the letters *a, b, c,* and so on as they are in the text citations (see 10.11, 10.25).

CROSS-REFERENCES

10.22   When a parenthetical reference in the text does not correspond exactly to the alphabetical listing of the source, a cross-reference may be necessary in the reference list (see 10.10, 11.2, and 12.2). Cross-references may also be used to shorten re-peated listings of the same book, such as a multiauthor book from which several authors' contributions are cited. If this method is used, begin the cross-reference with *in* rather than *see.* The examples below show parenthetical text citations fol-lowed by the corresponding reference list entries:

```
(Hay et al. 1975)
```

```
Hay, Douglas, Peter Linebaugh, John G. Rule, E. P.
    Thompson, and Cal Winslow. 1975. Albion's fatal
    tree: Crime and society in eighteenth-century
    England. New York: Pantheon.
```

```
(Hay 1975)
```

```
Hay, Douglas. 1975. Poaching and the game laws on
    Canning Chase. In Hay et al. 1975.
```

```
(Linebaugh 1975)
```

```
Linebaugh, Peter. 1975. The Tyburn riot against the
    surgeons. In Hay et al. 1975.
```

ARRANGEMENT OF ELEMENTS

10.23   In reference list entries the information elements are in the same order as in first, full note citations and bibliography en-tries (see 8.23–24, 9.7), except for the date (10.25). As in bibli-ographies, the elements are separated by periods, followed by a single space.

10.24   Reference list entries begin with the author's name, treated ex-actly as in bibliography entries (9.9–10).

10.25   For ease of locating an item in the reference list, the year of publication directly follows the author's name, as it does in the parenthetical reference in the text. If there is no date for a work or if it is still forthcoming, substitute *n.d.* (lowercase, not italicized) and place the work after others by the same author.

(Porkola 1990)

Porkola, Olga. 1990. *Contemporary Finnish design and architecture.* Cleveland: Cuyahoga Press.

(McGinnis n.d.)

McGinnis, J. P. n.d. *The surprising modernism of "Troilus and Cressida."* Forthcoming.

For periodicals the month, season, or day and month is also given, but following the name of the periodical. Seasons are not capitalized. In journal citations the season or month is enclosed in parentheses after the volume or issue number (there is no comma between the journal title and the volume number):

Hallinan, Maureen T., and Aage B. Sørensen. 1985. Class size, ability group size, and student achievement. *American Journal of Education* 94 (November): 71-89.

For magazines the season or month (or day and month) follows the name of the magazine but is not enclosed in parentheses. Instead, it is preceded by a comma and followed by a comma and the inclusive page numbers. (For the distinction between journals and magazines see 8.97.)

Karen, Robert. 1990. Becoming attached. *Atlantic,* February, 35-36.

In the author-date system, citations to items in daily newspapers are usually confined to the text, where they are treated somewhat as follows:

An editorial in the *Philadelphia Inquirer,* 30 June 1993, took the position that . . .

In an article titled "The Iron Curtain Goes Up," published in the *Wilberton Daily Journal,* 7 February 1990, Albert Finnonian reported that . . .

If it seems appropriate to include such citations in the reference list, the entries might be as follows:

Philadelphia Inquirer. 1993. Editorial, 30 June.

Finnonian, Albert. 1990. The Iron Curtain goes up. *Wilberton Daily Journal,* 7 February, final edition.

10.26   In the author-date system, the full titles and subtitles of books are capitalized sentence style (see 4.9) and italicized or underlined as titles are in notes.

> Slavin, Morris. 1984. *The French Revolution in miniature: "Section Droits-de-l'Homme," 1789–1795.* Princeton: Princeton University Press.

> Strier, Richard. 1983. *Love known: Theology and experience in George Herbert's poetry.* Chicago: University of Chicago Press.

10.27   The titles of series are capitalized headline style and not italicized or underlined:

> Charpentrat, Pierre. 1967. *L'art baroque.* Les Neuf Muses. Paris: Presses Universitaires de France.

> Creeley, Robert. 1970. *Quick graph: Collected notes and essays.* Edited by Donald Allen. Writing Series, no. 22. San Francisco: Four Seasons Foundation.

> Pollak, Ellen. 1985. *The poetics of sexual myth: Gender and ideology in the verse of Swift and Pope.* Women in Culture and Society. Chicago: University of Chicago Press.

10.28   The titles of chapters are capitalized sentence style with no quotation marks:

> McNeill, William H. 1976. The ecological impact of medical science and organization since 1700. Chapter 6 of *Plagues and peoples.* Garden City, N.Y.: Anchor/Doubleday.

10.29   The titles of periodical articles are capitalized sentence style with no quotation marks:

> Longstreth, Richard. 1985. From farm to campus: Planning, politics, and the agricultural college idea in Kansas. *Winterthur Portfolio* 20 (summer-autumn): 149–79.

10.30   In reference lists the titles of periodicals, both English language and foreign, are capitalized headline style and italicized or underlined as they are in notes (4.16). The names of professional journals may be abbreviated, using abbreviations accepted within the field of research:

> Chien Yu-chin and Barbara Lust. 1985. The concepts of topic and subject in first language acquisition of Mandarin Chinese. *Child Development* 56 (December): 1359–75.

Demsetz, Harold, and Kenneth Lehn. 1985. The structure of corporate ownership: Causes and consequences. *JPE* 93 (December): 1155-77.

Miller, Joanne, Kazimierz M. Slomczynski, and Melvin L. Kohn. 1985. Continuity of learning-generalization: The effect of job on men's intellective process in the United States and Poland. *AJS* 91 (November): 593-615.

10.31 Abbreviations are used for *edited by* (*ed.*), *translated by* (*trans.*), and *compiled by* (*comp.*), unless they might be misunderstood or unless they appear at the beginning of a segment in a reference list entry, when they are spelled out (see the last two examples below). Note that the editor follows, not precedes, the title of an edited book and is followed by the inclusive page numbers of the chapter cited (see 2.67)

Currie, David P. 1985. Sovereign immunity and suits against government officers. In *1984 Supreme Court Review,* ed. Philip W. Kurland, Gerhard Casper, and Dennis J. Hutchinson, 149-68. Chicago: University of Chicago Press.

Pollitt, Ernesto, Cutberto Garza, and Rudolph L. Leibel. 1984. Nutrition and public policy. In *Child development research and social policy,* ed. Harold W. Stevenson and Alberta E. Siegel, 1:421-70. Chicago: University of Chicago Press.

Derrida, Jacques. 1985. Racism's last word. Translated by Peggy Kamuf. *Critical Inquiry* 12 (autumn, special issue on "Race," Writing, and Difference): 290-99.

Ortega y Gasset, José. 1984. *Historical reason.* Translated by Philip W. Silver. New York: W. W. Norton.

10.32 With the exception of placing the year of publication after the name of the author, facts of publication in a reference list are given exactly as they would be given in a bibliography (see 9.11; and see also 8.52–69). For examples comparing parenthetical references and corresponding reference list entries with notes and bibliography entries for the same works, see chapters 11 and 12.

PARENTHETICAL REFERENCES USING NUMBERS

10.33 A related method of text reference gives only a number in the text: (9) or [9] or [9], as in some medical publications. This number refers not to a note but to an entry in a numbered list of works cited, placed at the end of the paper. This list may be arranged either alphabetically by authors' names or in order of appearance of each source in the text, as specified within the discipline governing the research. For guidelines recommended by particular fields in the physical and biological sciences, see the bibliography at the end of this manual.

10.34 In certain fields, principally the sciences, reference lists may follow a severely abbreviated style in which article titles are omitted and journal titles abbreviated. Consult the dissertation secretary or thesis adviser to determine whether the references in a paper should follow such a style and, if so, use an authoritative manual within the field.

11 Comparing the Two Documentation Systems

Books 11.3
    Single Author 11.3
    Two Authors 11.4
    Three Authors 11.5
    More Than Three Authors 11.6
    No Author Given 11.7
    No Author Given, Name Supplied 11.8
    Pseudonymous Author, Real Name Supplied 11.9
    Institution, Association, or the Like as "Author" 11.10
    Editor or Compiler as "Author" 11.11
    Author's Work Translated or Edited by Another 11.12
    Author's Work Contained in Collected Works 11.13
    Volume in a Multivolume Work with a General Title and
        Editor(s) 11.14
    Volume in a Multivolume Work with a General Title and
        One Author 11.15
    Book in a Series 11.16
    Book in a Series Naming the Series Editor 11.17
    Edition Other Than the First 11.18
    Reprint Edition 11.19
    Paperback Edition 11.20
    Title within a Title 11.21
    Book with Named Author of Introduction, Preface, or
        Foreword 11.24
    Book in a Foreign Language, Translation Supplied 11.25
    Component Part by One Author in a Work by Another
        11.26
    Component Part within a Work by One Author 11.27
    Complete Work within a Work by One Author 11.28
    Book Privately Printed 11.29
    Book Privately Printed, Publisher Not Known 11.30

Secondary Source of Quotation 11.31
Published Reports and Proceedings 11.32
  Published Reports 11.32
    Author Named 11.32
    Chairman of Committee Named 11.33
  Published Proceedings 11.34
    Author and Editor Named 11.34
    Article within Proceedings Published by an
      Institution, Association, or the Like 11.35
  Unpublished Reports and Proceedings 11.36
Yearbooks 11.37
  Department of Government 11.37
  Article in a Yearbook 11.38
Articles in Journals and Magazines 11.39
  Article in a Journal 11.39
  Article in a Magazine 11.41
Articles in Encyclopedias 11.42
  Unsigned Article 11.42
  Signed Article 11.43
Newspapers 11.44
Repeated References to Newspapers or Periodicals 11.45
Reviews 11.46
  Book Review in a Journal 11.46
  Unsigned Performance Review in a Newspaper 11.47
Interviews 11.48
  Published Interview 11.48
  Unpublished Interview 11.49
  Unpublished Interview by Writer of Paper 11.50
Microform Editions 11.51
Unpublished Materials 11.52
  Letter 11.52
  Speech 11.53
  Manuscript 11.54
  Thesis or Dissertation 11.55
  Material Obtained through an Information Service 11.56
  Electronic Document 11.57
Music 11.58
  Unpublished Musical Score 11.58
  Published Musical Score 11.59
Sound Recordings 11.60
Videorecordings 11.61
Performances 11.62

Works of Art 11.63
Works of Art Reproduced in Books 11.64
Multiple References within a Single Note 11.65

11.1 The following sets of examples illustrate note (N) and parenthetical reference (PR) forms and their corresponding bibliography (B) and reference list (RL) entries, except those used in citing public documents (for the latter, see chapter 12).

11.2 In a paper using parenthetical references keyed to a reference list, and even in some papers using notes and a bibliography, it may be useful to include cross-references for some citations. For example, it might be desirable to add a cross-reference in the reference list or bibliography for a work by a person who uses a pseudonym or for a work for which both the author and the writer of the foreword are listed. The choice of which name to cross-reference depends on the context within the paper, but the usage selected must be followed consistently. For the works listed below examples are included to illustrate any cross-references needed in the reference list (RL/CR) and the parenthetical text reference appropriate with each (PR/CR). Cross-references in bibliographies are the same as those in reference lists except for the dates. See also 10.10, 10.22, and 12.2.

BOOKS

SINGLE AUTHOR

11.3 N   [1]John Hope Franklin, *George Washington Williams: A Biography* (Chicago: University of Chicago Press, 1985), 54.

B   Franklin, John Hope. *George Washington Williams: A Biography*. Chicago: University of Chicago Press, 1985.

PR   (Franklin 1985, 54)

RL   Franklin, John Hope. 1985. *George Washington Williams: A biography*. Chicago: University of Chicago Press.

Two Authors

11.4   N   2. Robert Lynd and Helen Lynd, *Middletown:*
A Study in American Culture (New York:
Harcourt, Brace and World, 1929), 67.

     B   Lynd, Robert, and Helen Lynd. *Middletown: A*
Study in American Culture. New York:
Harcourt, Brace and World, 1929.

     PR   (Lynd and Lynd 1929, 67)

     RL   Lynd, Robert, and Helen Lynd. 1929. *Middletown:*
A study in American culture. New York:
Harcourt, Brace and World.

Three Authors

11.5   N   [3]Mary Lyon, Bryce Lyon, and Henry S.
Lucas, *The Wardrobe Book of William de Norwell,*
12 July 1338 to 27 May 1340, with the
collaboration of Jean de Sturler (Brussels:
Commission Royale d'Histoire de Belgique,
1983), 42.

     B   Lyon, Mary, Bryce Lyon, and Henry S. Lucas. *The*
Wardrobe Book of William de Norwell, 12
July 1338 to 27 May 1340. With the
collaboration of Jean de Sturler.
Brussels: Commission Royale d'Histoire de
Belgique, 1983.

     PR   (Lyon, Lyon, and Lucas 1983, 42)

     RL   Lyon, Mary, Bryce Lyon, and Henry S. Lucas.
1983. *The wardrobe book of William de*
Norwell, 12 July 1338 to 27 May 1340. With
the collaboration of Jean de Sturler.
Brussels: Commission Royale d'Histoire de
Belgique.

More Than Three Authors

11.6   N   4. Martin Greenberger and others, eds.,
Networks for Research and Education: Sharing of
Computer and Information Resources Nationwide
(Cambridge: MIT Press, 1974), 50.

     B   Greenberger, Martin, Julius Aronofsky, James L.
McKenney, and William F. Massy, eds.
Networks for Research and Education:
Sharing of Computer and Information

> *Resources Nationwide.* Cambridge: MIT Press, 1974.

PR   (Greenberger and others 1974, 50)

     or

     (Greenberger et al. 1974, 50)

RL   Greenberger, Martin, Julius Aronofsky, James L. McKenney, and William F. Massy, eds. 1974. *Networks for research and education: Sharing of computer and information resources nationwide.* Cambridge: MIT Press.

No Author Given

11.7 N   [5]*The Lottery* (London: J. Watts, [1732]), 20–25.

B   *The Lottery.* London: J. Watts, [1732].

PR   (*The lottery* [1732], 20–25)

RL   *The lottery.* [1732]. London: J. Watts.

No Author Given, Name Supplied

11.8 N   6. [Henry K. Blank], *Art for Its Own Sake* (Chicago: Nonpareil Press, 1910), 8.

B   [Blank, Henry K.]. *Art for Its Own Sake.* Chicago: Nonpareil Press, 1910.

PR   ([Blank] 1910, 8)

RL   [Blank, Henry K.]. 1910. *Art for its own sake.* Chicago: Nonpareil Press.

Pseudonymous Author, Real Name Supplied

11.9 See 8.27–30.

N   [7]Mrs. Markham, *A History of France* (London: John Murray, 1872), 9.

B   Markham, Mrs. [Elizabeth Cartright Penrose]. *A History of France.* London: John Murray, 1872.

PR   (Markham 1872, 9)

or

PR/CR   (Penrose 1872, 9)

RL   Markham, Mrs. [Elizabeth Cartright Penrose].
          1872. *A history of France*. London: John
          Murray.

RL/CR   Penrose, Elizabeth Cartright. 1872. *See*
          Markham, Mrs. [Elizabeth Cartright
          Penrose]. 1872.

INSTITUTION, ASSOCIATION, OR THE LIKE AS "AUTHOR"

11.10 N   8. American Library Association, Young
           Adult Services Division, Services Statement
           Development Committee, *Directions for Library
           Service to Young Adults* (Chicago: American
           Library Association, 1978), 25.

           B   American Library Association, Young Adult
                      Services Division, Services Statement
                      Development Committee. *Directions for
                      Library Service to Young Adults.* Chicago:
                      American Library Association, 1978.

           PR   (American Library Association 1978, 25)

           RL   American Library Association, Young Adult
                      Services Division, Services Statement
                      Development Committee. 1978. *Directions
                      for library service to young adults.*
                      Chicago: American Library Association.

EDITOR OR COMPILER AS "AUTHOR"

11.11 N   9Robert von Hallberg, ed., *Canons*
           (Chicago: University of Chicago Press, 1984),
           225.

           B   von Hallberg, Robert, ed. *Canons.* Chicago:
                      University of Chicago Press, 1984.

           PR   (von Hallberg 1984, 225)

           RL   von Hallberg, Robert, ed. 1984. *Canons.*
                      Chicago: University of Chicago Press.

AUTHOR'S WORK TRANSLATED OR EDITED BY ANOTHER

11.12 N   10. Jean Anouilh, *The Lark,* trans.
           Christopher Fry (London: Methuen, 1955), 86.

B	Anouilh, Jean. *The Lark.* Translated by Christopher Fry. London: Methuen, 1955.
PR	(Anouilh 1955, 86)
RL	Anouilh, Jean. 1955. *The lark.* Translated by Christopher Fry. London: Methuen.

AUTHOR'S WORK CONTAINED IN COLLECTED WORKS

11.13

N	[11]*The Complete Works of Samuel Taylor Coleridge,* ed. W. G. T. Shedd, vol. 1, *Aids to Reflection* (New York: Harper & Bros., 1884), 18.
B	Coleridge, Samuel Taylor. *The Complete Works of Samuel Taylor Coleridge.* Edited by W. G. T. Shedd. Vol. 1, *Aids to Reflection.* New York: Harper & Bros., 1884.
PR	(Coleridge 1884, 18)
RL	Coleridge, Samuel Taylor. 1884. *The complete works of Samuel Taylor Coleridge.* Edited by W. G. T. Shedd. Vol. 1, *Aids to reflection.* New York: Harper & Bros.

VOLUME IN A MULTIVOLUME WORK WITH A GENERAL TITLE AND EDITOR(S)

11.14

N	12. Gordon N. Ray, ed., *An Introduction to Literature,* vol. 2, *The Nature of Drama,* by Hubert Hefner (Boston: Houghton Mifflin, 1959), 47-49.
B	Ray, Gordon N., ed. *An Introduction to Literature.* Vol. 2, *The Nature of Drama,* by Hubert Hefner. Boston: Houghton Mifflin, 1959.
PR	(Ray 1959, 47-49)
	or
PR/CR	(Hefner 1959, 47-49)
RL	Ray, Gordon N., ed. 1959. *An introduction to literature.* Vol. 2, *The nature of drama,* by Hubert Hefner. Boston: Houghton Mifflin.
RL/CR	Hefner, Hubert. 1959. *See* Ray, Gordon N., ed. 1959.

See also 8.74.

VOLUME IN A MULTIVOLUME WORK WITH A GENERAL TITLE AND ONE AUTHOR

11.15 N   [13]Sewall Wright, *Evolution and the Genetics of Populations,* vol. 4, *Variability within and among Natural Populations* (Chicago: University of Chicago Press, 1978), 67.

  B   Wright, Sewall. *Evolution and the Genetics of Populations.* Vol. 4, *Variability within and among Natural Populations.* Chicago: University of Chicago Press, 1978.

  PR   (Wright 1978, 67)

  RL   Wright, Sewall. 1978. *Evolution and the genetics of populations.* Vol. 4, *Variability within and among natural populations.* Chicago: University of Chicago Press.

BOOK IN A SERIES

11.16 N   14. Ellen Pollak, *The Poetics of Sexual Myth: Gender and Ideology in the Verse of Swift and Pope,* Women in Culture and Society (Chicago: University of Chicago Press, 1985), 124.

  B   Pollak, Ellen. *The Poetics of Sexual Myth: Gender and Ideology in the Verse of Swift and Pope.* Women in Culture and Society. Chicago: University of Chicago Press, 1985.

  PR   (Pollak 1985, 124)

  RL   Pollak, Ellen. 1985. *The poetics of sexual myth: Gender and ideology in the verse of Swift and Pope.* Women in Culture and Society. Chicago: University of Chicago Press.

BOOKS IN A SERIES NAMING THE SERIES EDITOR

11.17 N   [15]Charles Issawi, *The Economic History of Turkey, 1800–1914,* Publications of the Center for Middle Eastern Studies, ed. Richard L. Chambers, no. 13 (Chicago: University of Chicago Press, 1980), 48.

B	Issawi, Charles. *The Economic History of Turkey, 1800-1914.* Publications of the Center for Middle Eastern Studies, ed. Richard L. Chambers, no. 13. Chicago: University of Chicago Press, 1980.
PR	(Issawi 1980, 48)
RL	Issawi, Charles. 1980. *The economic history of Turkey, 1800-1914.* Publications of the Center for Middle Eastern Studies, ed. Richard L. Chambers, no. 13. Chicago: University of Chicago Press.

EDITION OTHER THAN THE FIRST

11.18 Copyright pages often list successive printings or impressions, with the dates of each; note that these are not new *editions* of the book (see 8.45).

N	16. M. M. Bober, *Karl Marx's Interpretation of History,* 2d ed. Harvard Economic Studies (Cambridge: Harvard University Press, 1948), 89.
B	Bober, M. M. *Karl Marx's Interpretation of History,* 2d ed. Harvard Economic Studies. Cambridge: Harvard University Press, 1948.
PR	(Bober 1948, 89)
RL	Bober, M. M. 1948. *Karl Marx's interpretation of history.* 2d ed. Harvard Economic Studies. Cambridge: Harvard University Press.

REPRINT EDITION

11.19 In notes the publisher and date of a reprint edition are given following the usual information about the book as originally issued. In reference list entries the date of the source the citation was taken from follows the author's name, and the date and publisher of the original edition are added either following the title or at the end of the entry as shown below:

N	[17]Michael David, *Toward Honesty in Public Relations* (Chicago: Condor Publications, 1968; reprint, New York: B. Y. Jove, 1990), 134-56 (page citations are to the reprint edition).
B	David, Michael. *Toward Honesty in Public*

        Relations. Chicago: Condor Publications, 1968. Reprint, New York: B. Y. Jove, 1990.

PR   (David 1990, 134-56)

RL   David, Michael. 1990. *Toward honesty in public relations.* Chicago: Condor Publications, 1968. Reprint, New York: B. Y. Jove (page references are to the reprint edition).

        or

        David, Michael. 1990. *Toward honesty in public relations.* New York: B. Y. Jove. Original edition, Chicago: Condor Publications, 1968.

Paperback Edition

11.20   Entries for paperback reprints should also give original publication data as well as reprint data; citations of original paperbacks often are identified by the name of the paperback line (e.g., Anchor Books, Phoenix Books):

N   18. George F. Kennan, *American Diplomacy, 1900-1950* (Chicago: University of Chicago Press, 1951; Phoenix Books, 1970), 50.

B   Kennan, George F. *American Diplomacy, 1900-1950.* Chicago: University of Chicago Press, 1951; Phoenix Books, 1970.

PR   (Kennan 1970, 50)

RL   Kennan, George F. 1970. *American diplomacy, 1900-1950.* Chicago: University of Chicago Press, 1951. Reprint, Phoenix Books (page references are to the reprint edition).

        or

        Kennan, George F. 1970. *American diplomacy, 1900-1950.* Chicago: University of Chicago Press, Phoenix Books. Original edition, Chicago: University of Chicago Press, 1951.

Title within a Title

11.21   A title of another work that would itself ordinarily be italicized or underlined is enclosed in double quotation marks when it appears as part of an italicized title:

N   [19]Allen Forte, *The Harmonic Organization of
         "The Rite of Spring"* (New Haven: Yale
         University Press, 1978), 50.

B   Forte, Allen. *The Harmonic Organization of "The
             Rite of Spring."* New Haven: Yale
             University Press, 1978.

PR   (Forte 1978, 50)

RL   Forte, Allen. 1978. *The harmonic organization
             of "The rite of spring."* New Haven: Yale
             University Press.

11.22   When the title of a book occurs within the title of a journal
         article, poem, or short story, whether the latter is in quotation
         marks or not (as in a reference list), the book title is italicized
         or underlined:

N   20. Carl Avren Levenson, "Distance and
         Presence in Augustine's *Confessions*," *Journal
         of Religion* 65 (October 1985): 508, n. 4.

B   Levenson, Carl Avren. "Distance and Presence in
             Augustine's *Confessions*." *Journal of
             Religion* 65 (October 1985): 500–512.

PR   (Levenson 1985, 508, n. 4)

RL   Levenson, Carl Avren. 1985. Distance and
             presence in Augustine's *Confessions*.
             Journal of Religion 65 (October): 500–512.

11.23   When the title of an article appears within the title of another
         article, single quotation marks are used:

         "Comment on 'How to Make a Burden of the Public Debt'"

Book with Named Author of Introduction, Preface, or Foreword

11.24 N   [21]Dag Hammarskjöld, *Markings,* with a
         foreword by W. H. Auden (New York: Alfred A.
         Knopf, 1964), 10.

B   Hammarskjöld, Dag. *Markings.* With a foreword by
             W. H. Auden. New York: Alfred A. Knopf,
             1964.

PR   (Hammarskjöld 1964, 10)

RL   Hammarskjöld, Dag. 1964. *Markings.* With a
             foreword by W. H. Auden. New York: Alfred
             A. Knopf.

If Auden's authorship of the foreword was more significant than Hammarskjöld's book in the context of a paper citing this work, the following would be the correct form:

N   22. W. H. Auden, foreword to *Markings,* by Dag Hammarskjöld (New York: Alfred A. Knopf, 1964), ix.

B   Auden, W. H. Foreword to *Markings,* by Dag Hammarskjöld. New York: Alfred A. Knopf, 1964.

PR   (Auden 1964, ix)

RL   Auden, W. H. 1964. Foreword to *Markings,* by Dag Hammarskjöld. New York: Alfred A. Knopf.

BOOK IN A FOREIGN LANGUAGE, TRANSLATION SUPPLIED

11.25   N   [23]Martin Buber, *Das Problem des Menschen* (The problem of man) (Heidelberg: Lambert Scheider Verlag, 1948), 35.

B   Buber, Martin. *Das Problem des Menschen* (The problem of man). Heidelberg: Lambert Scheider Verlag, 1948.

PR   (Buber 1948, 35)

RL   Buber, Martin. 1948. *Das Problem des Menschen* (The problem of man). Heidelberg: Lambert Scheider Verlag.

Note that the translation of the title and its subtitle, if any, is neither italicized nor put in quotation marks but is put in parentheses and capitalized sentence style.

COMPONENT PART BY ONE AUTHOR IN A WORK BY ANOTHER

11.26   N   24. Mary Higdon Beech, "The Domestic Realm in the Lives of Hindu Women in Calcutta," in *Separate Worlds: Studies of Purdah in South Asia,* ed. Hanna Papanek and Gail Minault (Delhi: Chanakya, 1982), 115.

B   Beech, Mary Higdon. "The Domestic Realm in the Lives of Hindu Women in Calcutta." In *Separate Worlds: Studies of purdah in South Asia,* ed. Hanna Papnanek and Gail Minault, 110-38. Delhi: Chanakya, 1982.

PR   (Beech 1982, 115)

RL   Beech, Mary Higdon. 1982. The domestic realm in
the lives of Hindu women in Calcutta. In
*Separate worlds: Studies of purdah in
South Asia,* ed. Hanna Papanek and Gail
Minault, 110-38. Delhi: Chanakya.

Component Part within a Work by One Author

11.27 N   [25]Bruno Bettelheim, "The Frame Story of
Thousand and One Nights," in *The Uses of
Enchantment: The Meaning and Importance of
Fairy Tales* (New York: Vintage Books, 1976),
87.

      B   Bettelheim, Bruno. "The Frame Story of *Thousand
and One Nights."* In *The Uses of
Enchantment: The Meaning and Importance of
Fairy Tales.* New York: Vintage Books,
1976.

     PR   (Bettelheim 1976, 87)

     RL   Bettelheim, Bruno. 1976. The frame story of
Thousand and one nights. In *The uses of
enchantment: The meaning and importance of
fairy tales.* New York: Vintage Books.

Complete Work within a Work by One Author

11.28   Titles of short poems and short stories should be put in double
quotation marks, but italicize or underline the titles of longer
works.

     N   26. John Milton, *Paradise Lost,* in *The
Complete Poetical Works of John Milton,* ed.
William Vaughn Moody, Student's Cambridge
Edition (Boston: Houghton Mifflin, 1899), 102.

     B   Milton, John. *Paradise Lost.* In *The Complete
Poetical Works of John Milton,* ed. William
Vaughn Moody. Student's Cambridge Edition.
Boston: Houghton Mifflin, 1899.

     PR   (Milton 1899, 102).

     RL   Milton, John. 1899. *Paradise lost.* In *The
complete poetical works of John Milton,*
ed. William Vaughn Moody. Student's
Cambridge Edition. Boston: Houghton
Mifflin.

11.29 / Comparing the Two Documentation Systems

BOOK PRIVATELY PRINTED

11.29 N   [27]John G. Barrow, *A Bibliography of Bibliographies in Religion* (Austin, Tex.: by the author, 1955), 25.

B   Barrow, John G. *A Bibliography of Bibliographies in Religion.* Austin, Tex.: by the author, 1955.

PR   (Barrow 1955, 25)

RL   Barrow, John G. 1955. *A bibliography of bibliographies in religion.* Austin, Tex.: by the author.

BOOK PRIVATELY PRINTED, PUBLISHER NOT KNOWN

11.30 N   28. Frank Budgen, *Further Recollections of James Joyce* (London: privately printed, 1955), 10.

B   Budgen, Frank. *Further Recollections of James Joyce.* London: privately printed, 1955.

PR   (Budgen 1955, 10)

RL   Budgen, Frank. 1955. *Further recollections of James Joyce.* London: privately printed.

SECONDARY SOURCE OF QUOTATION

11.31 N   [29]Roland Barthes, "La mort de l'auteur" (The death of the author), *Manteia,* vol. 5 (1968); trans. Stephen Heath in *Image/Music/Text* (New York: Hill and Wang, 1977), 147; quoted in Wayne C. Booth, *Critical Understanding: The Powers and Limits of Pluralism* (Chicago: University of Chicago Press, 1979), 372-73, n. 9.

B   Barthes, Roland. "La mort de l'auteur" (The death of the author). *Manteia,* vol. 5 (1968). Translated by Stephen Heath in *Image/Music/Text.* New York: Hill and Wang, 1977, 147. Quoted in Wayne C. Booth, *Critical Understanding: The Powers and Limits of Pluralism,* 372-73, n. 9. Chicago: University of Chicago Press, 1979.

PR   (Barthes 1968)

RL   Barthes, Roland. 1968. "La mort de l'auteur"
      (The death of the author). *Manteia,* vol.
      5. Translated by Stephen Heath in *Image/*
      music/text. New York: Hill and Wang, 1977,
      147. Quoted in Wayne C. Booth. *Critical*
      understanding: The powers and limits of
      pluralism, 372-73, n. 9. Chicago:
      University of Chicago Press, 1979.

PUBLISHED REPORTS AND PROCEEDINGS

PUBLISHED REPORTS

11.32 *Author named*

N   30. B. G. F. Cohen, *Human Aspects in*
      Office Automation (Cincinnati: National
      Institute for Occupational Safety and Health,
      Division of Biomedical and Behavioral Science,
      1984), 150, NTIS, PB84-240738.

B   Cohen, B. G. F. *Human Aspects in Office*
          Automation. Cincinnati: National Institute
          for Occupational Safety and Health,
          Division of Biomedical and Behavioral
          Science, 1984. NTIS, PB84-240738.

PR   (Cohen 1984, 150)

RL   Cohen, B. G. F. 1984. *Human aspects in office*
          automation. Cincinnati: National Institute
          for Occupational Safety and Health,
          Division of Biomedical and Behavioral
          Science. NTIS, PB84-240738.

11.33 *Chairman of committee named*

N   [31]*Report of the Committee on Financial*
      Institutions to the President of the United
      States, by Walter W. Heller, chairman
      (Washington, D.C.: Government Printing Office,
      1963), 12.

B   *Report of the Committee on Financial*
          Institutions to the President of the
          United States. By Walter W. Heller,
          chairman. Washington, D.C.: Government
          Printing Office, 1963.

PR   (*Report of the Committee on Financial*
      Institutions 1963, 12)

            or

PR/CR (Heller 1963, 12)

RL   *Report of the Committee on Financial*

> *Institutions to the President of the*
> *United States. 1963. By Walter W. Heller,*
> chairman. Washington, D.C.: Government
> Printing Office.

RL/CR   Heller, Walter W. 1963. See *Report of the*
> *Committee on Financial Institutions. 1963.*

PUBLISHED PROCEEDINGS

11.34   *Author and editor named*

N   32. S. Akazawa, "The Scope of the Japanese
> Information Industry in the 1980s," in *The*
> *Challenge of Information Technology:*
> *Proceedings of the Forty-first FID (Fédération*
> *Internationale de Documentation) Congress Held*
> *in Hong Kong 13-16 September 1982,* ed. K. R.
> Brown (Amsterdam, New York, and Oxford: North-
> Holland, 1983), 20.

B   Akazawa, S. "The Scope of the Japanese
> Information Industry in the 1980s." In *The*
> *Challenge of Information Technology:*
> *Proceedings of the Forty-first FID*
> *(Fédération Internationale de*
> *Documentation) Congress Held in Hong Kong*
> *13-16 September 1982,* edited by K. R.
> Brown, 19-22. Amsterdam, New York, and
> Oxford: North-Holland, 1983.

PR   (Akazawa 1983, 20)

RL   Akazawa, S. 1983. The scope of the Japanese
> information industry in the 1980s. In *The*
> *challenge of information technology:*
> *Proceedings of the forty-first FID*
> *(Fédération Internationale de*
> *Documentation) congress held in Hong Kong*
> *13-16 September 1982,* edited by K. R.
> Brown, 19-22. Amsterdam, New York, and
> Oxford: North-Holland.

11.35   *Article within proceedings published by an institution, associa-*
tion, or the like

N   [33]Pere Martin Oelberg, "Norway and Latin
> American Development," in *Latin American-*
> *European Business Cooperation: Proceedings of*
> *the Symposium in Montreaux, Switzerland,*
> *November 20-22, 1979,* by the Inter-American
> Development Bank (Switzerland: Inter-American
> Development Bank, 1979), 81.

B   Oelberg, Pere Martin. "Norway and Latin
> American Development." In *Latin American-*

200

European Business Cooperation: Proceedings
of the Symposium in Montreaux,
Switzerland, November 20-22, 1979, by the
Inter-American Development Bank, 80-83.
Switzerland: Inter-American Development
Bank, 1979.

PR   (Oelberg 1979, 81)

RL   Oelberg, Pere Martin. 1979. Norway and Latin
American development. In *Latin American-
European business cooperation: Proceedings
of the symposium in Montreaux,
Switzerland, November 20-22, 1979,* by the
Inter-American Development Bank, 80-83.
Switzerland: Inter-American Development
Bank.

UNPUBLISHED REPORTS AND PROCEEDINGS

11.36   Titles of unpublished reports and proceedings are put in quotation marks. When not given in the title, place and date follow the title. There may also be the notation "typewritten" or "photocopied."

N   34. George Psacharopoulos and Keith
Hincliffe, "Tracer Study Guidelines"
(Washington, D.C.: World Bank, Education
Department, 1983, photocopied), 5.

B   Psacharopoulos, George, and Keith Hincliffe.
"Tracer Study Guidelines." Washington,
D.C.: World Bank, Education Department,
1983. Photocopied.

PR   (Psacharopoulos and Hincliffe 1983, 5)

RL   Psacharopoulos, George, and Keith Hincliffe.
1983. Tracer study guidelines. Washington,
D.C.: World Bank, Education Department.
Photocopied.

YEARBOOKS

DEPARTMENT OF GOVERNMENT

11.37   N   [35]U.S. Department of Agriculture, *Will
There Be Enough Food? The 1981 Yearbook of
Agriculture* (Washington, D.C.: Government
Printing Office, 1981), 250.

B   U.S. Department of Agriculture. *Will There Be*

> *Enough Food? The 1981 Yearbook of Agriculture.* Washington, D.C.: Government Printing Office, 1981.

PR   (U.S. Department of Agriculture 1981, 250)

RL   U.S. Department of Agriculture. 1981. *Will there be enough food? The 1981 yearbook of agriculture.* Washington, D.C.: Government Printing Office.

ARTICLE IN A YEARBOOK

11.38 N   36. G. M. Wilson, "A Survey of the Social Business Use of Arithmetic," in *Sixteenth Yearbook of the National Society for the Study of Education* (Bloomington, Ill.: Public School Publishing Co., 1917), 21.

  B   Wilson, G. M. "A Survey of the Social Business Use of Arithmetic." In *Sixteenth Yearbook of the National Society for the Study of Education,* 20-22. Bloomington, Ill.: Public School Publishing Co., 1917.

  PR   (Wilson 1917, 21)

  RL   Wilson, G. M. 1917. A survey of the social business use of arithmetic. In *Sixteenth yearbook of the National Society for the Study of Education,* 20-22. Bloomington, Ill.: Public School Publishing Co.

ARTICLES IN JOURNALS AND MAGAZINES

ARTICLE IN A JOURNAL

11.39 N   [37]Richard Jackson, "Running down the Up-Escalator: Regional Inequality in Papua New Guinea," *Australian Geographer* 14 (May 1979): 180.

  B   Jackson, Richard. "Running down the Up-Escalator: Regional Inequality in Papua New Guinea." *Australian Geographer* 14 (May 1979): 175-84.

  PR   (Jackson 1979, 180)

  RL   Jackson, Richard. 1979. Running down the up-escalator: Regional inequality in Papua New Guinea. *Australian Geographer* 14 (May): 175-84.

11.40   For citing journals that are numbered only by issue, or by volume and issue, note the style shown in 8.101. For citing journals that publish volumes in successive numbered or lettered series, see 8.102.

N   38. Lawrence P. Smith, "Sailing Close to the Wind," *Politics in Action* 10, no. 4 (1993): 82, 99–100.

B   Smith, Lawrence P. "Sailing Close to the Wind." *Politics in Action* 10, no. 4 (1993): 80–102.

PR   (Smith 1993, 82, 99–100)

RL   Smith, Lawrence P. 1993. Sailing close to the wind. *Politics in Action* 10, no. 4:80–102.

N   ³⁹R. Broom and J. T. Robinson, "Man Contemporaneous with the Swartkrans Ape-Man," *American Journal of Physical Anthropology,* n.s., 8 (1950): 154.

B   Broom, R., and J. T. Robinson. "Man Contemporaneous with the Swartkrans Ape-Man." *American Journal of Physical Anthropology,* n.s., 8 (1950): 151–56.

PR   (Broom and Robinson 1950, 154)

RL   Broom, R., and J. T. Robinson. 1950. Man contemporaneous with the Swartkrans ape-man. *American Journal of Physical Anthropology,* n.s., 8:151–56.

ARTICLE IN A MAGAZINE

11.41   N   40. Bruce Weber, "The Myth Maker: The Creative Mind of Novelist E. L. Doctorow," *New York Times Magazine,* 20 October 1985, 42.

B   Weber, Bruce. "The Myth Maker: The Creative Mind of Novelist E. L. Doctorow." *New York Times Magazine,* 20 October 1985, 42.

PR   (Weber 1985, 42)

RL   Weber, Bruce. 1985. The myth maker: The creative mind of novelist E. L. Doctorow. *New York Times Magazine,* 20 October, 42.

See also 8.71.

ARTICLES IN ENCYCLOPEDIAS

UNSIGNED ARTICLE

11.42   Well-known reference books are generally not listed in bibliographies. In notes or parenthetical references the facts of publication are usually omitted, but the edition, if not the first, must be specified (see 8.112):

N   [41]*Columbia Encyclopedia,* 5th ed., s.v. "cold war."

PR   (*Columbia Encyclopedia,* 5th ed., s.v. "cold war")

SIGNED ARTICLE

11.43   If the article is signed, the author's name may be included:

N   42. Morris Jastrow, "Nebo," in *Encyclopaedia Britannica,* 11th ed.

PR   (Morris Jastrow, "Nebo," in *Encyclopaedia Britannica,* 11th ed.)

NEWSPAPERS

11.44   News items from daily papers are rarely listed separately in a bibliography or reference list. If a newspaper is cited only once or twice, a note or a parenthetical reference in the text is sufficient:

N   [43]*Irish Daily Independent* (Dublin), 16 June 1904.

PR   (*Irish Daily Independent* [Dublin], 16 June 1904).

Several matters to be considered in referring to newspapers are discussed in 8.105–10.

REPEATED REFERENCES TO NEWSPAPERS OR PERIODICALS

11.45   If the writer has used issues of a newspaper or periodical covering a considerable period, this fact may be indicated by giving the title of the publication plus the dates. Such references are usually grouped in a separate section of the bibliography or reference list:

B   *Times* (London). 4 January–6 June 1964.

RL   *Times* (London). 1964. 4 January–6 June.

B   *Saturday Review.* 2, 16, 30 July; 2, 20, 27
          August 1966.

RL   *Saturday Review.* 1966. 2, 16, 30 July; 2, 20,
          27 August.

REVIEWS

BOOK REVIEW IN A JOURNAL

11.46 N   [45]Dwight Frankfather, review of *The
                    Disabled State,* by Deborah A. Stone, *Social
                    Service Review* 59 (September 1985): 524.

         B   Frankfather, Dwight. Review of *The Disabled
                    State,* by Deborah A. Stone. *Social Service
                    Review* 59 (September 1985): 523–25.

         PR   (Frankfather 1985, 524)

         RL   Frankfather, Dwight. 1985. Review of *The
                    disabled state,* by Deborah A. Stone.
                    Social Service Review 59 (September): 523–
                    25.

Citations of reviews of films and performances in a journal follow the same style.

UNSIGNED PERFORMANCE REVIEW IN A NEWSPAPER

11.47 Citations of reviews of plays, films, and musical performances published in newspapers or weekly magazines also follow the same style, though reference to a location is customary only in a drama review.

         N   46. Review of *Fool for Love,* by Sam
                    Shepard (Circle Repertory Company, New York),
                    New York Times, 27 May 1983, 18(N) and C3(L).

         B   Review of *Fool for Love,* by Sam Shepard. Circle
                    Repertory Company, New York. *New York
                    Times,* 27 May 1983, 18(N) and C3(L).

      PR   (Review of *Fool for love* 1983, 18[N])

      RL   Review of *Fool for love,* by Sam Shepard. 1983. Circle Repertory Company, New York. *New York Times,* 27 May, 18(N) and C3(L).

INTERVIEWS

PUBLISHED INTERVIEW

11.48 N   [47]John Fowles, "A Conversation with John Fowles," interview by Robert Foulke (Lyme Regis, 3 April 1984), *Salmagundi,* nos. 68-69 (fall 1985-winter 1986): 370.

      B   Fowles, John. "A Conversation with John Fowles." Interview by Robert Foulke (Lyme Regis, 3 April 1984). *Salmagundi,* nos. 68-69 (fall 1985-winter 1986): 367-84.

      PR   (Fowles 1985-86, 370)

      RL   Fowles, John. 1985-86. A conversation with John Fowles. Interview by Robert Foulke (Lyme Regis, 3 April 1984). *Salmagundi,* nos. 68-69 (fall-winter): 367-84.

UNPUBLISHED INTERVIEW

11.49 N   48. Benjamin Spock, interview by Milton J. E. Senn, 20 November 1974, interview 67A, transcript, Senn Oral History Collection, National Library of Medicine, Bethesda, Md.

      B   Spock, Benjamin. Interview by Milton J. E. Senn, 20 November 1974. Interview 67A, transcript. Senn Oral History Collection, National Library of Medicine, Bethesda, Md.

      PR   (Spock 1974)

      RL   Spock, Benjamin. 1974. Interview by Milton J. E. Senn, 20 November. Interview 67A, transcript. Senn Oral History Collection, National Library of Medicine, Bethesda, Md.

UNPUBLISHED INTERVIEW BY WRITER OF PAPER

11.50 N   [49]Mayor Harold Washington of Chicago, interview by author, 23 September 1985,

Chicago, tape recording, Chicago Historical
Society, Chicago.

B   Washington, Harold, mayor of Chicago. Interview
by author, 23 September 1985, Chicago.
Tape recording. Chicago Historical
Society, Chicago.

PR   (Washington 1985)

RL   Washington, Harold, mayor of Chicago. 1985.
Interview by author, 23 September,
Chicago. Tape recording. Chicago
Historical Society, Chicago.

MICROFORM EDITIONS

11.51 N   50. William Voelke, ed., *Masterpieces of
Medieval Painting: The Art of Illumination*
(Pierpont Morgan Library, New York; Chicago:
University of Chicago Press, 1980), text-fiche,
p. 56, 4F6-4F10.

B   Voelke, William, ed. *Masterpieces of Medieval
Painting: The Art of Illumination.*
Pierpont Morgan Library, New York;
Chicago: University of Chicago Press,
1980. Text-fiche.

PR   (Voelke 1980, p. 56, 4F6-4F10)

RL   Voelke, William, ed. 1980. *Masterpieces of
medieval painting: The art of
illumination.* Pierpont Morgan Library, New
York; Chicago: University of Chicago
Press. Text-fiche.

UNPUBLISHED MATERIALS

LETTER

11.52 N   [51]Percy Bysshe Shelley, Padua, to Mary
Wollstonecraft Shelley, Este, 22 September
1818, transcript in the hand of Mary
Wollstonecraft Shelley, Special Collections,
Joseph Regenstein Library, University of
Chicago, Chicago.

B   Shelley, Percy Bysshe, Padua, to Mary
Wollstonecraft Shelley, Este, 22 September
1818. Transcript in the hand of Mary
Wollstonecraft Shelley. Special

Collections, Joseph Regenstein Library,
University of Chicago, Chicago.

PR   (Shelley 1818)

RL   Shelley, Percy Bysshe. 1818. Letter from Padua
        to Mary Wollstonecraft Shelley, Este, 22
        September. Transcript in the hand of Mary
        Wollstonecraft Shelley. Special
        Collections, Joseph Regenstein Library,
        University of Chicago, Chicago.

See also 2.19 for abbreviations used to describe manuscripts
and 8.131–32.

SPEECH

11.53 N   52. Eulogy of Charles V in Latin,
        apparently written at the monastery of St.
        Just, Spain, [ca. 1500], Special Collections,
        Joseph Regenstein Library, University of
        Chicago, Chicago.

B   Eulogy of Charles V. In Latin, apparently
        written at the monastery of St. Just,
        Spain, [ca. 1500]. Special Collections,
        Joseph Regenstein Library, University of
        Chicago, Chicago.

PR   (Eulogy of Charles V [ca. 1500])

RL   Eulogy of Charles V. [Ca. 1500.] In Latin,
        apparently written at the monastery of St.
        Just, Spain. Special Collections, Joseph
        Regenstein Library, University of Chicago,
        Chicago.

MANUSCRIPT

11.54 N   [53]Robert Craft, "A Catalog of Manuscripts
        and Documents [of] the Original Works of Igor
        Stravinsky, 1970(?)," TMs (photocopy), p. 136,
        Special Collections, Joseph Regenstein Library,
        University of Chicago, Chicago.

B   Craft, Robert. "A Catalog of Manuscripts and
        Documents [of] the Original Works of Igor
        Stravinsky, 1970(?)." TMs (photocopy).
        Special Collections, Joseph Regenstein
        Library, University of Chicago, Chicago.

PR   (Craft 1970[?], 136)

RL   Craft, Robert. 1970(?). A catalog of
manuscripts and documents [of] the
original works of Igor Stravinsky. TMs
(photocopy). Special Collections, Joseph
Regenstein Library, University of Chicago,
Chicago.

The use of the question mark in parentheses after the date
means that its accuracy is uncertain, even though parts of the
manuscript may have been dated with some certainty. Note
that if an unpublished manuscript is undated but a reliable date
has been supplied, this date appears in brackets (see 8.68).
Brackets are also used in place of parentheses within parentheses.

THESIS OR DISSERTATION

11.55 N   54. Gilberto Artioli, "Structural Studies
of the Water Molecules and Hydrogen Bonding in
Zeolites" (Ph.D. diss., University of Chicago,
1985), 10.

      B   Artioli, Gilberto. "Structural Studies of the
Water Molecules and Hydrogen Bonding in
Zeolites." Ph.D. diss., University of
Chicago, 1985.

      PR   (Artioli 1985, 10)

      RL   Artioli, Gilberto. 1985. Structural studies of
the water molecules and hydrogen bonding
in zeolites. Ph.D. diss., University of
Chicago.

MATERIAL OBTAINED THROUGH AN INFORMATION SERVICE

11.56 N   [55]Susan J. Kupisch, *Stepping In,* paper
presented as part of the symposium "Disrupted
and Reorganized Families" at the annual meeting
of the Southeastern Psychological Association,
Atlanta, Ga., 23–26 March 1983, Dialog, ERIC,
ED 233 276.

      B   Kupisch, Susan J. *Stepping In.* Paper presented
as part of the symposium "Disrupted and
Reorganized Families" at the annual
meeting of the Southeastern Psychological
Association, Atlanta, Ga., 23–26 March
1983. Dialog, ERIC, ED 233 276.

      PR   (Kupisch 1983)

RL Kupisch, Susan J. 1983. *Stepping in.* Paper presented as part of the symposium "Disrupted and reorganized families" at the annual meeting of the Southeastern Psychological Association, Atlanta, Ga., 23–26 March. Dialog, ERIC, ED 233 276.

See also 8.139 and 12.20.

ELECTRONIC DOCUMENT

11.57 N 56. Rosabel Flax, *Guidelines for Teaching Mathematics K-12* (Topeka: Kansas State Department of Education, 1979) [database on-line]; available from Dialog, ERIC, ED 178312.

   B Flax, Rosabel. *Guidelines for Teaching Mathematics K-12.* Topeka: Kansas Department of Education, 1979. Database on-line. Available from Dialog, ERIC, ED 178312.

   PR (Flax 1979)

   RL Flax, Rosabel. 1979. *Guidelines for teaching mathematics K-12.* Topeka: Kansas Department of Education. Database on-line. Available from Dialog, ERIC, ED 178312.

MUSIC

UNPUBLISHED MUSICAL SCORE

11.58 N [57]Ralph Shapey, "Partita for Violin and Thirteen Players," score, 1966, Special Collections, Joseph Regenstein Library, University of Chicago, Chicago.

   B Shapey, Ralph. "Partita for Violin and Thirteen Players." Score. 1966. Special Collections, Joseph Regenstein Library, University of Chicago, Chicago.

   PR (Shapey 1966)

   RL Shapey, Ralph. 1966. Partita for violin and thirteen players. Score. Special Collections, Joseph Regenstein Library, University of Chicago, Chicago.

PUBLISHED MUSICAL SCORE

11.59 N 58. Wolfgang Amadeus Mozart, *Don Giovanni,* libretto by Lorenzo da Ponte, English version

by W. H. Auden and Chester Kallman (New York
and London: G. Schirmer, 1961), 55.

B   Mozart, Wolfgang Amadeus. *Don Giovanni.*
        Libretto by Lorenzo da Ponte, English
        version by W. H. Auden and Chester
        Kallman. New York and London: G. Schirmer,
        1961.

PR   (Mozart 1961, 55)

RL   Mozart, Wolfgang Amadeus. 1961. *Don Giovanni.*
        Libretto by Lorenzo da Ponte, English
        version by W. H. Auden and Chester
        Kallman. New York and London: G.
        Schirmer.

SOUND RECORDINGS

11.60 N   [59]Norman Mailer, *The Naked and the Dead,*
excerpts read by the author, Caedmon CP1619,
1983, cassette.

B   Mailer, Norman. *The Naked and the Dead.*
        Excerpts read by the author. Caedmon
        CP1619, 1983. Cassette.

PR   (Mailer 1983)

RL   Mailer, Norman. 1983. *The naked and the dead.*
        Excerpts read by the author. Caedmon
        CP1619. Cassette.

VIDEORECORDINGS

11.61 N   60. *Itzak Perlman: In My Case Music,* prod.
and dir. Tony DeNonno, 10 min., DeNonno Pix,
1985, videocassette.

B   Perlman, Itzak. *Itzak Perlman: In My Case
        Music.* Produced and directed by Tony
        DeNonno. 10 min. DeNonno Pix, 1985.
        Videocassette.

PR   (Perlman 1985)

RL   Perlman, Itzak. 1985. *Itzak Perlman: In my case
        music.* Produced and directed by Tony
        DeNonno. 10 min. DeNonno Pix.
        Videocassette.

PERFORMANCES

11.62 N   [61]William Shakespeare, *The Winter's Tale,* Festival Theatre, Stratford, Ontario, 24 September 1986.

      B   Shakespeare, William. *The Winter's Tale.* Festival Theatre, Stratford, Ontario, 24 September 1986.

      PR   (Shakespeare 1986)

      RL   Shakespeare, William. 1986. *The winter's tale.* Festival Theatre, Stratford, Ontario, 24 September.

WORKS OF ART

11.63   Actual works of art are normally not included in a bibliography or reference list. They may be described in a note or a parenthetical reference in the text (see 8.147):

      N   62. Jackson Pollock, *Reflection of the Big Dipper,* oil on canvas, 1946, Stedelijk Museum, Amsterdam.

      PR   (Jackson Pollock, *Reflection of the Big Dipper,* oil on canvas, 1946, Stedlijk Museum, Amsterdam)

WORKS OF ART REPRODUCED IN BOOKS

11.64   References to reproductions of works of art in published sources are treated much like citations of a chapter or other component part of a book:

      N   [63]Thomas Nast, "The Tammany Tiger Loose: 'What Are You Going to Do about It,'" cartoon, *Harper's Weekly,* 11 November 1871, as reproduced in J. Chal Vinson, *Thomas Nast: Political Cartoonist* (Athens: University of Georgia Press, 1967), plate 52.

      B   Nast, Thomas. "The Tammany Tiger Loose: 'What Are You Going to Do about It.'" Cartoon. *Harper's Weekly,* 11 November 1871. As reproduced in J. Chal Vinson, *Thomas Nast: Political Cartoonist,* plate 52. Athens: University of Georgia Press, 1967.

      PR   (Nast 1967, plate 52)

RL   Nast, Thomas. 1967. The Tammany tiger loose:
      "What are you going to do about it."
      Cartoon. *Harper's Weekly,* 11 November
      1871. As reproduced in J. Chal Vinson,
      Thomas Nast: Political cartoonist, plate
      52. Athens: University of Georgia Press.

MULTIPLE REFERENCES WITHIN A SINGLE NOTE

11.65 The individual references in a note citing several works are
separated by semicolons and listed in the order in which they
were cited:

> 64. See Samuel P. Langley, *James Smithson*
> (Washington, D.C.: Smithsonian Institution, 1904), 18-
> 19; Paul Oehser, *Sons of Science* (New York: Henry
> Schuman, 1949), 1, 9-11; and Webster True, *The First
> Hundred Years of the Smithsonian Institution, 1846-1946*
> (Washington, D.C.: Smithsonian Institution, 1946), 2-
> 106.

11.66 The bibliography entries for multiple references in a single note
must, of course, be alphabetized separately:

> Langley, Samuel P. *James Smithson*. Washington, D.C.:
>   Smithsonian Institution, 1904.
>
> Oehser, Paul. *Sons of Science.* New York: Henry
>   Schuman, 1949.
>
> True, Webster. *The First Hundred Years of the
>   Smithsonian Institution, 1846-1946.* Washington,
>   D.C.: Smithsonian Institution, 1946.

11.67 In papers using parenthetical references, the multiple citations
appear as follows:

> (Langley 1904, 18-19; Oehser 1949, 1, 9-11; True 1946,
> 2-106)

11.68 A reference list entry must be included for each author:

> Langley, Samuel P. 1904. *James Smithson*. Washington,
>   D.C.: Smithsonian Institution.
>
> Oehser, Paul. 1949. *Sons of science.* New York: Henry
>   Schuman.
>
> True, Webster. 1946. *The first hundred years of the
>   Smithsonian Institution, 1846-1946.* Washington,
>   D.C.: Smithsonian Institution.

12 Public Documents

Form of Citations 12.3
United States Government Documents 12.5
    Published Documents 12.8
        Legislative Publications 12.8
            Hearings 12.9
            Bills and Resolutions 12.10
            Debates 12.12
        Presidential Documents 12.13
        United States Constitution 12.15
        Publications by Government Commissions 12.16
        Executive Department Documents 12.17
        Treaties 12.18
    Unpublished Documents 12.19
    Technical Reports 12.20
State and Local Government Documents 12.21
British Government Documents 12.22
    Parliamentary Papers 12.26
    Sessional Papers 12.27
    Parliamentary Debates 12.28
    British Foreign and State Papers 12.29
Canadian Public Documents 12.32
Documents of International Bodies 12.33

12.1   Before research for a paper begins, consideration should be given to the proper form for citations to public documents, so that full bibliographical data can be gathered from printed, microfilmed, televised, or on-line materials at the time they are being examined. For example, all citations to on-line materials must include identifying numbers within the information services. All dates of publication must be recorded. While conducting research for a paper that includes a reference list, it is also a good idea to record any abbreviations and authors' names that will have to be cross-referenced.

12.2   In papers using author-date citations, it is often useful to cite the issuing agency rather than the government responsible for the work, which should be the first item in a reference list entry. For this reason the reference list may need a number of cross-references. For example, the parenthetical reference "(U.S. Congress 1941)" is adequate if a reference list includes only one such entry. If there are both Senate and House entries for 1941, however, the parenthetical reference should read "(U.S. Congress, House 1941)." Sometimes a document is known by its title or by the name of the committee of the Senate or House that drafted it. In that case a parenthetical reference keyed to the first item in the reference list entry, "(U.S. Congress 1941)," for example, would not be as useful as one keyed to a cross-reference in the reference list. For example, the parenthetical reference "(*Declarations of a state of war with Japan, Germany, and Italy* 1941)" must be keyed to a cross-reference in the reference list that reads "*Declarations of a state of war with Japan, Germany, and Italy.* 1941. *See* U.S. Congress. 1941." In referring to the source within the text, use either a parenthetical reference (PR) keyed to the full citation in the reference list (RL) or a parenthetical cross-reference (PR/CR) keyed to a cross-reference in the reference list (RL/CR), and do one or the other consistently for a particular item. The full citation in the reference list is the same whether a parenthetical reference or a parenthetical cross-reference is used. The examples in this chapter also include samples of notes (N) and corresponding bibliography entries (B).

FORM OF CITATIONS

12.3   The form used for citing public documents should make them readily accessible to anyone wishing to locate them in standard indexes, information services, and libraries. The arrangement of information on the title pages of the documents themselves, its amount, and its complexity raise puzzling questions of how much of it one must include and in what order within a note, bibliography entry, or reference list entry. Here the card catalog of the library can be of great assistance, although it is not a safe guide in such matters as capitalization and punctuation of titles, which must follow the scheme of the paper. When in doubt about how much to include in a reference, it is better to give too much information than too little.

12.4 The name of the country, state, city, town, or other government district (e.g., U.S., U.K. [United Kingdom], Illinois, Baltimore) is given first in the citation of an official publication issued by one of these or under its auspices. Unlike bibliography or reference list entries, note references to public documents need not begin with the name of the country unless it is not obvious from the text. Next comes the name of the legislative body, court, executive department, bureau, board, commission, or committee. The name of the office rather than the title of the officer should be given except where that title is the only name of the office, as, for example, "Illinois, State Entomologist." The name of any division, regional office, or the like, follows the name of the department, bureau, or commission. Thus the "author" of a document might read: "U.S., Department of Labor, Manpower Administration, Office of Manpower Policy and Research." Following the name of the author, the title of the document, if any, should be given, in italics or underlined, capitalized headline style in notes and bibliographies and sentence style in reference lists. From this point the information included depends largely on the nature of the material.

UNITED STATES GOVERNMENT DOCUMENTS

12.5 The United States government publishes its official documents in two main categories, originating in Congress or in the executive departments. Publications are issued by both houses (Senate and House of Representatives), by the executive departments (State, Justice, Labor, etc.), and by agencies (Federal Trade Commission, General Services Administration, etc.). In addition to these, the *Monthly Catalog of United States Government Publications* also lists an array of technical reports: government-sponsored research, development, and engineering reports and foreign technical reports and other analyses prepared by national and local government agencies and by their contractors or grantees. Many of these materials are available through such information services as the National Technical Information Service (NTIS) and the Educational

Resources Information Center (ERIC) (see 12.20). Their proliferation requires that the information in citations to public documents include all available facts of publication (dates, serial and print numbers, etc.) as well as information service identifying and accession numbers when available.

12.6   For citations to government publications, use one of the following styles consistently throughout a paper:

```
Washington, D.C.: U.S. Government Printing Office,
   1980.
Washington, D.C.: Government Printing Office, 1980.
Washington, D.C.: GPO, 1980.
Washington, D.C., 1980
Washington, 1980.
```

12.7   The *Congressional Information Service Index* (*CIS/Index*) provides current comprehensive coverage of committee hearings, House and Senate reports and documents, Senate executive reports, and Senate treaty documents. This information may be accessed through printed serial volumes and microfiches available at depository libraries or through several large computer services. The proceedings of each house of Congress, together with the presidential messages to it, are published at the close of each legislative day. Citations to all such hearings, reports, and documents must include—in addition to the authorizing body—the number, session, and date of the Congress; title and number (if any) of the document; and in some instances, the title of the work in which the document can be found, with relevant volume and page number(s).

PUBLISHED DOCUMENTS

LEGISLATIVE PUBLICATIONS

12.8   N

```
        [2]House Committee on Interior and Insular
        Affairs, Subcommittee on Energy and the
        Environment, International Proliferation of
        Nuclear Technology, report prepared by Warren
        H. Donnelley and Barbara Rather, 94th Cong., 2d
        sess., 1976, Committee Print 15, 5.
```

B

```
        U.S. Congress. House. Committee on Interior and
        Insular Affairs. Subcommittee on Energy
        and the Environment. International
        Proliferation of Nuclear Technology.
        Report prepared by Warren H. Donnelley and
```

Barbara Rather. 94th Cong., 2d sess., 1976. Committee Print 15.

PR   (U.S. Congress, House 1976, 5)

          or

PR/CR   (Donnelley and Rather 1976, 5)

          or

PR/CR   (*International proliferation of nuclear technology* 1976, 5)

RL   U.S. Congress. House. Committee on Interior and Insular Affairs. Subcommittee on Energy and the Environment. 1976. *International proliferation of nuclear technology.* Report prepared by Warren H. Donnelley and Barbara Rather. 94th Cong., 2d sess. Committee Print 15.

RL/CR   Donnelley and Rather. 1976. *See* U.S. Congress. House. 1976.

          or

RL/CR   *International proliferation of nuclear technology.* 1976. *See* U.S. Congress. House. 1976.

N   [2]House, *A Bill to Require Passenger-Carrying Motor Vehicles Purchased for Use by the Federal Government to Meet Certain Safety Standards,* 86th Cong., 1st sess., 1959, H.R. 1341, 8.

B   U.S. Congress. House. *A Bill to Require Passenger-Carrying Motor Vehicles Purchased for Use by the Federal Government to Meet Certain Safety Standards.* 86th Cong., 1st sess., 1959. H.R. 1341.

PR   (U.S. Congress, House 1959, 8)

RL   U.S. Congress. House. 1959. *A bill to require passenger-carrying motor vehicles purchased for use by the federal government to meet certain safety standards.* 86th Cong., 1st sess. H.R. 1341.

N   [3]Congress, *Declarations of a State of War with Japan, Germany, and Italy,* 77th Cong., 1st sess., 1941, S. Doc. 148, Serial 10575.

B   U.S. Congress. *Declarations of a State of War with Japan, Germany, and Italy.* 77th Cong., 1st sess., 1941. S. Doc. 148. Serial 10575.

PR   (U.S. Congress 1941)

        or

PR/CR (*Declarations of a state of war* 1941)

RL   U.S. Congress. 1941. *Declarations of a state of war with Japan, Germany, and Italy.* 77th Cong., 1st sess. S. Doc. 148. Serial 10575.

RL/CR *Declarations of a state of war.* 1941. *See* U.S. Congress. 1941.

N   [3]Congress, Senate, Committee on Foreign Relations, *U.S. Scholarship Program for Developing Countries* (Washington, D.C.: GPO, 1984), 7.

B   U.S. Congress. Senate. Committee on Foreign Relations. *U.S. Scholarship Program for Developing Countries.* Washington, D.C.: GPO, 1984.

PR   (U.S. Congress, Senate 1984, 7)

RL   U.S. Congress. Senate. Committee on Foreign Relations. 1984. *U.S. scholarship program for developing countries.* Washington, D.C.: GPO.

12.9   *Hearings.* Hearings should be cited by title. Even if the "author" listed on the publication does not indicate the committee before which the hearings were held, the committee should be named as the "author" in the reference:

N   1. Congress, Senate, Committee on Foreign Relations, *Famine in Africa: Hearing before the Committee on Foreign Relations,* 99th Cong., 1st sess., 17 January 1985, 57.

B   U.S. Congress. Senate. Committee on Foreign Relations. *Famine in Africa: Hearing before the Committee on Foreign Relations.* 99th Cong., 1st sess., 17 January 1985.

PR   (U.S. Congress, Senate 1985, 57)

RL   U.S. Congress. Senate. Committee on Foreign Relations. 1985. *Famine in Africa: Hearing*

> *before the Committee on Foreign Relations.*
> 99th Cong., 1st sess., 17 January.

12.10 *Bills and resolutions.* Congressional bills (proposed laws) and resolutions are published in pamphlet form (slip bills) and are available on microfiche at many libraries. When a bill is enacted into law, it becomes part of the *Statutes at Large.* In the interim between its being introduced into one of the houses and its passage and publication as a law in the *Statutes* (see 12.11), a bill is cited to a slip bill or to the *Congressional Record:*

N
    ²Congress, House, *Food Security Act of 1985,* 99th Cong., 1st sess., H.R. 2100, *Congressional Record,* 131, no. 132, daily ed. (8 October 1985): H8485.

B
    U.S. Congress. House. *Food Security Act of 1985.* 99th Cong., 1st sess., H.R. 2100. *Congressional Record.* 131, no. 132, daily ed. (8 October 1985): H8353-H8486.

PR
    (U.S. Congress, House 1985, H8485)

    or

PR/CR
    (*Food Security Act of 1985,* H8485)

RL
    U.S. Congress. House. 1985. *Food Security Act of 1985.* 99th Cong., 1st sess., H.R. 2100. *Congressional Record,* 131, no. 132, daily ed. (8 October): H8353-H8486.

RL/CR
    Food Security Act of 1985. See U.S. Congress. House. 1985.

12.11 After their passage, bills and joint resolutions are cited as statutes. Statutes are published in the *United States Statutes at Large* issued for the year during which they have gone into effect (sample note 13 below). Later, the statutes are incorporated into the *United States Code* (note 14).

N
    13. *Administrative Procedure Act, Statutes at Large* 60, sec. 10, 243 (1946).

B
    Administrative Procedure Act. Statutes at Large 60 (1946).

PR
    (*Administrative Procedure Act* 1946)

RL
    Administrative Procedure Act. Statutes at large. 1946. Vol. 60, sec. 10, 243.

N
    14. *Declaratory Judgment Act, U.S. Code,* vol. 28, secs. 2201-2 (1952).

B   *Declaratory Judgment Act. U.S. Code.* Vol. 28, secs. 2201-2 (1952).

PR   (*Declaratory Judgment Act* 1952)

RL   *Declaratory Judgment Act. U.S. Code.* 1952. Vol. 28, secs. 2201-2.

Citations to the *Code* are always to section number, not page.

12.12   *Debates.* Congressional debates are printed in the *Congressional Record.* Unless the subject of the speech or remarks is mentioned in the text, it is proper to include it in the citation. This example refers to the bound volume, which often contains material revised since its appearance in the *Daily Digest* and is paged differently.

N   [3]Congress, Senate, Senator Kennedy of Massachusetts speaking for the Joint Resolution on Nuclear Weapons Freeze and Reductions to the Committee on Foreign Relations, S.J. Res. 163, 97th Cong., 1st sess., *Congressional Record* 128, pt. 3 (10 March 1982): 3832-34

B   U.S. Congress. Senate. Senator Kennedy of Massachusetts speaking for the Joint Resolution on Nuclear Weapons Freeze and Reductions to the Committee on Foreign Relations. S.J. Res. 163. 97th Cong., 1st sess. *Congressional Record* 128, pt. 3 (10 March 1982).

PR   (U.S. Congress, Senate 1982, 3832-34)

RL   U.S. Congress. Senate. 1982. Senator Kennedy of Massachusetts speaking for the Joint Resolution on Nuclear Weapons Freeze and Reductions to the Committee on Foreign Relations. S.J. Res. 163. 97th Cong., 1st sess. *Congressional Record* 128, pt. 3 (10 March).

PRESIDENTIAL DOCUMENTS

12.13   *The Weekly Compilation of Presidential Documents* publishes in serial form presidential proclamations, executive orders, and such other documents as addresses, letters, and vetoes. Presidential proclamations and executive orders are also carried in the *Federal Register,* published daily.

N   4. President, Proclamation, "Caribbean

Basin Economic Recovery Act, Proclamation 5142,
Amending Proclamation 5133," *Federal Register*
49, no. 2 (4 January 1984): 341, microfiche.

B   U.S. President. Proclamation. "Caribbean Basin
        Economic Recovery Act, Proclamation 5142,
        Amending Proclamation 5133." *Federal
        Register* 49, no. 2 (4 January 1984): 341.
        Microfiche.

PR   (U.S. President 1984, 341)

RL   U.S. President. 1984. Proclamation. Caribbean
        Basin Economic Recovery Act, Proclamation
        5142, amending Proclamation 5133. *Federal
        Register* 49, no. 2 (4 January): 341.
        Microfiche.

12.14 The public papers of the presidents of the United States are
collected in two large multivolume works.

N   [11]J. D. Richardson, ed., *Compilation of the
        Messages and Papers of the Presidents, 1789-
        1897,* 53d Cong., 2d sess., 1907, *House
        Miscellaneous Document no. 210* (Washington,
        D.C.: Government Printing Office, 1907), 4:16.

B   Richardson, J. D., ed. *Compilation of the
        Messages and Papers of the Presidents,
        1789-1897.* 53d Cong., 2d sess., 1907,
        House Miscellaneous Document no. 210. Pts.
        1-10, 10 vols. Washington, D.C.:
        Government Printing Office, 1907.

PR   (Richardson 1907, 4:16)

RL   Richardson, J. D., ed. 1907. *Compilation of the
        messages and papers of the presidents,
        1789-1897.* 53d Cong., 2d sess., *House
        miscellaneous document no. 210.* Pts. 1-10,
        10 vols. Washington, D.C.: Government
        Printing Office.

N   [12]U.S. President, *Public Papers of the
        Presidents of the United States* (Washington,
        D.C.: Office of the *Federal Register,* National
        Archives and Records Service, 1956), Dwight D.
        Eisenhower, 1956, 222-23.

B   U.S. President. *Public Papers of the Presidents
        of the United States.* Washington, D.C.:
        Office of the *Federal Register,* National
        Archives and Records Service, 1953-.
        Dwight D. Eisenhower, 1956.

PR   (U.S. President 1956, 222-23)

RL   U.S. President. 1956. *Public papers of the presidents of the United States.* Washington, D.C.: Office of the *Federal Register,* National Archives and Records Service, 1953-. Dwight D. Eisenhower.

UNITED STATES CONSTITUTION

12.15   The United States Constitution is cited by article or amendment, section, and, if relevant, clause. Abbreviations and arabic numerals are used in referring to all parts of the document (see also 2.27). Citations to the Constitution are usually given in the text or notes. It is unnecessary to list the Constitution in the bibliography or reference list.

[16]U.S. Constitution, art. 1, sec. 4.

[17]U.S. Constitution, amend. 14, sec. 2.

PUBLICATIONS BY GOVERNMENT COMMISSIONS

12.16   Several government commissions, such as the Federal Communications Commission, Federal Trade Commission, and Securities and Exchange Commission, also publish bulletins, circulars, reports, study papers, and the like. These are often classified as House or Senate documents.

N   1. Securities and Exchange Commission, *Annual Report of the Securities and Exchange Commission for the Fiscal Year* (Washington, D.C.: GPO, 1983), 42.

B   U.S. Securities and Exchange Commission. *Annual Report of the Securities and Exchange Commission for the Fiscal Year.* Washington, D.C.: GPO, 1983.

PR   (U.S. Securities and Exchange Commission 1983, 42)

RL   U.S. Securities and Exchange Commission. 1983. *Annual report of the Securities and Exchange Commission for the fiscal year.* Washington, D.C.: GPO.

N   2. Congress, Senate, *Report of the Federal Trade Commission on Utility Corporations,* 70th Cong., 1st sess., 1935, S. Doc. 91, pt. 71A.

B   U.S. Congress. Senate. *Report of the Federal

> Trade Commission on Utility Corporations. 70th Cong., 1st sess., 1935. S. Doc. 91, pt. 71A.

PR   (U.S. Congress 1935)

RL   U.S. Congress. Senate. 1935. *Report of the Federal Trade Commission on utility corporations.* 70th Cong., 1st sess., S. Doc. 91, pt. 71A.

EXECUTIVE DEPARTMENT DOCUMENTS

12.17   Executive department documents consist of reports, bulletins, circulars, and miscellaneous materials issued by executive departments, bureaus, and agencies. When authors of these publications are identified, they should be included in the citations along with the issuing body. The citation usually begins with the name of the issuing body, but it may also begin with the name of the author. When both are included in the bibliography entry, one should be cross-referenced to the other.

N   [1]Department of the Interior, Minerals Management Service, *An Oilspill Risk Analysis for the Central Gulf (April 1984) and Western Gulf of Mexico (July 1984),* by Robert P. LaBelle, open-file report, U.S. Geological Survey, 83-119 (Denver, 1983), lease offerings microfilm.

B   U.S. Department of the Interior. Minerals Management Service. *An Oilspill Risk Analysis for the Central Gulf (April 1984) and Western Gulf of Mexico (July 1984),* by Robert P. LaBelle. Open-file report, U.S. Geological Survey. Denver, 1983. Lease offerings microfilm.

PR   (U.S. Department of the Interior 1983)

or

PR/CR   (LaBelle 1983)

RL   U.S. Department of the Interior. Minerals Management Service. 1983. *An oilspill risk analysis for the central Gulf (April 1984) and western Gulf of Mexico (July 1984),* by Robert P. LaBelle. Open-file report, U.S. Geological Survey, 83-119. Denver. Lease offerings microfilm.

RL/CR   LaBelle, Robert P. 1983. *See* U.S. Department of the Interior. 1983.

N   ⁴Department of Labor, Employment Standards Administration, *Resource Book: Training for Federal Employee Compensation Specialists* (Washington, D.C., 1984), 236.

B   U.S. Department of Labor. Employment Standards Administration. *Resource Book: Training for Federal Employee Compensation Specialists.* Washington, D.C., 1984.

PR   (U.S. Department of Labor 1984, 236)

RL   U.S. Department of Labor. Employment Standards Administration. 1984. *Resource book: Training for federal employee compensation specialists.* Washington, D.C.

TREATIES

12.18 Since 1950, treaties have been published in the annual bound volumes of *United States Treaties and Other International Agreements.* The treaties appear in these bound volumes as they were numbered and published in pamphlet form by the Department of State in the series Treaties and Other International Acts (TIAS). Multilateral treaties, those involving more than two countries, appear in the Treaty Series of the United Nations, but usually not until a year or more after their signing. Depending on their nature and date, treaties predating 1950 may be found in one or another of the following: Treaty Series of the League of Nations, Treaty Series and Executive Agreement Series of the Department of State, and *Statutes at Large.*

N   8. Department of State, "Nuclear Weapons Test Ban," 5 August 1963, TIAS no. 5433, *United States Treaties and Other International Agreements,* vol. 14, pt. 2.

B   U.S. Department of State. "Nuclear Weapons Test Ban," 5 August 1963. TIAS no. 5433. *United States Treaties and Other International Agreements,* vol. 14, pt. 2.

PR   (U.S. Department of State 1963)

RL   U.S. Department of State. 1963. Nuclear Weapons Test Ban, 5 August 1963. TIAS no. 5433. *United States treaties and other international agreements,* vol. 14, pt. 2.

N   9. U.S., "Naval Armament Limitation

Treaty," 26 February 1922, *Statutes at Large,*
(December 1923-March 1925), vol. 43, pt. 2.

B   U.S. "Naval Armament Limitation Treaty," 26
        February 1922. *Statutes at Large* (December
        1923-March 1925), vol. 43, pt. 2.

PR   (U.S. 1922)

RL   U.S. 1922. Naval Armament Limitation Treaty, 26
        February 1922. *Statutes at large* (December
        1923-March 1925), vol. 43, pt. 2.

N   10. "Denmark and Italy: Convention
        concerning Military Service," 15 July 1954,
        *Treaties and International Agreements
        Registered or Filed or Reported with the
        Secretariat of the United Nations* 250, no. 3516
        (1956): 45.

B   United Nations. Treaty Series. "Denmark and
        Italy: Convention concerning Military
        Service," 15 July 1954. *Treaties and
        International Agreements Registered or
        Filed or Reported with the Secretariat of
        the United Nations,* 250 (1956), no. 3516.

PR   (United Nations, Treaty Series 1956, 250, no.
        3516:45)

RL   United Nations. Treaty Series. 1956. Denmark
        and Italy: Convention concerning military
        service, 15 July 1954. *Treaties and
        international agreements registered or
        filed or reported with the Secretariat of
        the United Nations,* 250, no. 3516.

Unpublished Documents

12.19   Most unpublished documents of the United States government
are held in the National Archives in Washington, D.C., or in
one of its branches. All materials, including manuscripts and
typescript records, films, still photographs, and sound recordings, are cited by record group (RG) number. They may
also have titles and file numbers, which should be included in
any citation. *The Chicago Manual of Style,* fourteenth edition
(15.374–75, 16.176) gives suggestions for ordering the information in citations to such materials. For papers involving many
citations to unpublished public documents, use the method of
citation below. The style adopted should be applied consis-

tently throughout the notes and bibliography or parenthetical references and reference list.

N   ²Senate Committee on the Judiciary,
           "Lobbying," file 71A-F15, RG 46, National
           Archives.

B   U.S. Congress. Senate. Committee on the
           Judiciary. "Lobbying." File 71A-F15. RG
           46. National Archives.

PR   (U.S. Congress, Senate n.d.)

           or

PR/CR   (Lobbying n.d.)

RL   U.S. Congress. Senate. Committee on the
           Judiciary. n.d. Lobbying. File 71A-F15. RG
           46. National Archives.

RL/CR   Lobbying. n.d. *See* U.S. Congress. Senate. n.d.

TECHNICAL REPORTS

12.20   Under the category of United States public documents falls an extensive collection of technical reports readily available through large information services, several of which can be accessed through such computer services as Dialog and Orbit. Many of these reports stem from contracts and grants awarded by federal agencies to universities, specialized consultants, corporations, and professional associations and societies. The National Technical Information Service (NTIS), a federal agency within the Department of Commerce, provides copies of scientific and technical reports produced by federal agencies and their contractors and recovers the costs of this service from sales to users. NTIS distributes many government and nongovernment printed materials that are not sent to depository libraries. It also tracks the scientific and technical material available through depository library networks. Another such large information network is the Educational Resources Information Center (ERIC), which makes available education-related materials. For an excellent discussion of technical report literature, its background, and current availability, see chapter 5 of *Introduction to United States Public Documents,* by Joe Morehead, available at the reference desks of most research libraries. Much of the information from these services is available on-line, on paper, or on microfiche. The following examples show how to refer to several kinds of technical reports:

N   8. Barbara Robson, *Tanzania: Country Status Report* (Washington, D.C.: Center for Applied Linguistics, Language/Area Reference Center, 1984), 7, ERIC, ED 248700.

B   Robson, Barbara. *Tanzania: Country Status Report*. Washington, D.C.: Center for Applied Linguistics, Language/Area Reference Center, 1984. ERIC, ED 248700.

PR   (Robson 1984, 7)

RL   Robson, Barbara. 1984. *Tanzania: Country status report*. Washington, D.C.: Center for Applied Linguistics, Language/Area Reference Center. ERIC, ED 248700.

N   9. *Act of 18 March 1983 on Nuclear Third Party Liability (LRCN)* (Paris: French Government, 1983), 6, NTIS, DE84780322.

B   *Act of 18 March 1983 on Nuclear Third Party Liability (LRCN)*. Paris: French Government, 1983. NTIS, DE84780322.

PR   (*Act of 18 March* 1983, 6)

           or

PR/CR   (Nuclear Third Party Liability Act 1983, 6)

RL   *Act of 18 March 1983 on Nuclear Third Party Liability (LRCN)*. 1983. Paris: French Government. NTIS, DE84780322.

RL/CR   Nuclear Third Party Liability Act. 1983. See *Act of 18 March 1983 on Nuclear Third Party Liability*. 1983.

N   10. Bureau of Intelligence and Research, *Indicators of Comparative East-West Economic Strength, 1981,* by L. Kornei, 7 December 1982, 5, NTIS, AD-A145 450/3.

B   U.S. Bureau of Intelligence and Research. *Indicators of Comparative East-West Economic Strength, 1981*. By L. Kornei. 7 December 1982. NTIS, AD-A145 450/3.

PR   (U.S. Bureau of Intelligence and Research 1982, 5)

           or

PR/CR   (Kornei 1982, 5)

RL   U.S. Bureau of Intelligence and Research.
*Indicators of comparative East-West
economic strength, 1981.* By L. Kornei. 7
December. NTIS, AD-A145 450/3.

RL/CR   Kornei, L. 1982. *See* U.S. Bureau of
Intelligence and Research. 1982.

N   11. Stephanie R. Peters and Neil C.
Silverstein, "Predicting Success in Graduate
School," paper presented at the annual meeting
of the American Educational Research
Association, Seattle, Wash., 21-24 April 1995
[database on-line]; available from DIALOG,
ERIC, ED 685923.

B   Peters, Stephanie R., and Neil C. Silverstein.
"Predicting Success in Graduate School."
Paper presented at the annual meeting of
the American Educational Research
Association, Seattle, Wash., 21-24 April
1995. Database on-line. Available from
DIALOG, ERIC, ED 685923.

PR   (Peters and Silverstein 1995)

RL   Peters, Stephanie R., and Neil C. Silverstein.
1995. Predicting success in graduate
school. Paper presented at the annual
meeting of the American Educational
Research Association, Seattle, Wash., 21-
24 April. Database on-line. Available from
DIALOG, ERIC, ED 685923.

STATE AND LOCAL GOVERNMENT DOCUMENTS

12.21   Citations to state and local government documents take essentially the same form as those to United States government documents:

N   [1]Illinois Constitution (1848), art. 5,
sec. 2.

Ordinarily, the date of a constitution is given only when it is not in force. In papers using the author-date system, constitutional citations are usually given in the text, and it is unnecessary to include constitutional entries in either bibliographies or reference lists. Note 2 below shows the style used in referring to an annotated revision made by William K. Baldwin in 1943.

N   [2]*Revised Statutes, Annotated* (Baldwin,
1943).

B   Kentucky. *Revised Statutes, Annotated* (Baldwin, 1943).

PR   (Kentucky 1943)

RL   Kentucky. 1943. *Revised statutes, annotated* (Baldwin).

N   [3]Ohio, *Judicial Organization Act, Statutes* (1830), 3:1571-78.

B   Ohio. *Judicial Organization Act. Statutes.* 1830.

PR   (Ohio 1830, 3:1571-78)

RL   Ohio. 1830. *Judicial Organization Act. Statutes.*

N   [4]New York, N.Y., *"Good Samaritan" Law, Administrative Code* (1965), sec. 67-3.2.

B   New York, N.Y. *"Good Samaritan" Law. Administrative Code.* 1965.

PR   (New York 1965, sec. 67-3.2)

          or

PR/CR (*"Good Samaritan" law* 1965, sec. 67-3.2)

RL   New York, N.Y. 1965. *"Good Samaritan" law. Administrative code.*

RL/CR *"Good Samaritan" law.* 1965. *See* New York, N.Y. 1965.

BRITISH GOVERNMENT DOCUMENTS

12.22   Citations to British government documents, like those to their United States counterparts, should begin with the name of the authorizing body—Parliament, Public Record Office, Foreign Office, Ministry of Transport, and so on—always preceded by "United Kingdom" (if published since 1801) or "Great Britain" (if published between 1707 and 1801) or "England" if dated before 1707).

12.23   *Anglo-American Cataloguing Rules* has recommended that British government publications be listed under United Kingdom (sometimes abbreviated U.K.), although Great Britain (abbreviated G.B.) was widely used until recently and is also acceptable, taking into consideration the dates of publication involved (see 12.22).

12.24 The publisher of most British government material in recent years is Her (His) Majesty's Stationery Office (HMSO) in London.

12.25 More often cited in notes or text than in bibliographies or reference lists, English statutes are always cited by title (not in italic or underlined), regnal year of the sovereign (for those passed before 1963) or year (for those passed since 1963), and chapter (c.) number (arabic numerals for national statutes, roman numerals for local). Listing the titles of statutes passed before the 1850s may present difficulties, because shortened titles of acts were not always designated, as they have been by law since 1892. In the second set of examples below, for instance, the document is simply described in place of a title. In references to English statutes passed before 1963, names of sovereigns are abbreviated and arabic numerals are used for regnal year (tables of regnal years are available in many reference works). Since 1963 published statutes have been numbered serially within each calendar year, so these statutes are cited by year and chapter number. Before publication in the *Statutes* or in the *Public General Acts and Church Assembly Measures* (called the *Public General Acts and General Synod Measures* since 1972), statutes are cited as in the first set of examples below. When they are published in one compilation or the other, their citations follow the forms shown in the last two sets.

N   1. Laws, Statutes, etc., *Coroner's Act, 1954*, 2 & 3 Eliz. 2, c. 31.

B   United Kingdom. [*or* U.K.]. Laws, Statutes, etc. *Coroner's Act, 1954*. 2 & 3 Eliz. 2, c. 31.

PR   (United Kingdom. Laws, Statutes, etc. 1954)

         or

PR/CR   (*Coroner's Act* 1954)

RL   United Kingdom. Laws, Statutes, etc. 1954. *Coroner's Act, 1954*. 2 & 3 Eliz. 2, c. 31.

RL/CR   *Coroner's Act*. 1954. *See* United Kingdom. Laws, Statutes, etc. 1954.

N   2. King's General Pardon, 1540, *Statutes of the Realm*, 32 Hen. 8, c. 49.

B   England. King's General Pardon. 1540. *Statutes of the Realm.* 32 Hen. 8, c. 49.

PR   (England, King's General Pardon 1540)

     or

PR   (England 1540)

RL   England. King's General Pardon. 1540. *Statutes of the Realm.* 32 Hen. 8, c. 49.

N   3. *Statutes,* 31 Vict., c. xiv, 2 April 1868.

B   United Kingdom. *Statutes.* 31 Vict., c. xiv. 2 April 1868.

PR   (United Kingdom 1868)

RL   United Kingdom. 1868. *Statutes.* 31 Vict., c. xiv. 2 April.

N   4. Laws, Statutes, etc., *Police and Criminal Evidence Act, 1984, Public General Acts and General Synod Measures,* 1984, pt. 3, c. 60.

B   United Kingdom. Laws, Statutes, etc. *Police and Criminal Evidence Act, 1984. Public General Acts and General Synod Measures,* 1984, pt. 3, c. 60.

PR   (United Kingdom. Laws, Statutes, etc. 1984)

RL   United Kingdom. Laws, Statutes, etc. 1984. *Police and Criminal Evidence Act, 1984. Public General Acts and General Synod Measures,* pt. 3, c. 60.

PARLIAMENTARY PAPERS

12.26 The Parliamentary Papers are bound annually in two sequences, each with its own series of volume numbers. In one sequence public acts are arranged alphabetically by the official names of the acts, with related committee proceedings and reports following each bill. In the other sequence reports, accounts, and papers (sometimes called Sessional Papers) are arranged alphabetically by primary subject matter. The *Sessional Index* is a useful guide to pagination and organization within these two sequences. Among the Parliamentary Papers discussed above are "command papers," so named because they are presented by command of the reigning monarch. For numbering and abbreviations for consecutive series of command papers, see *The Chicago Manual of Style,* fourteenth edition (15.395, 16.184). The term *parliamentary papers* also refers to such other publications of the House of Commons and the House of Lords as their journals, votes, proceedings, and debates (see 12.28).

N   [7]*Report of the Royal Commission on Indian Currency and Finance,* vol. 2, Appendices, Cmd. 2687 (1926).

B   United Kingdom. *Report of the Royal Commission on Indian Currency and Finance.* Vol. 2, Appendices. Cmd. 2687. 1926.

PR   (United Kingdom 1926)

RL   United Kingdom. 1926. *Report of the Royal Commission on Indian Currency and Finance.* Vol. 2, Appendices. Cmd. 2687.

N   [8]The *Basle Facility and the Sterling Area,* Cmnd. 3787 (October 1968), 15-16.

B   United Kingdom. *The Basle Facility and the Sterling Area.* Cmnd. 3787. October 1968.

PR   (United Kingdom 1968, 15-16)

RL   United Kingdom. 1968. *The Basle facility and the Sterling area.* Cmnd. 3787. October.

SESSIONAL PAPERS

12.27   The Sessional Papers are a part of the Parliamentary Papers, but the latter are also sometimes referred to as Sessional Papers. Though the annual series of Sessional Papers is identified by year date alone, it is divided into titles, each title having its individual set of volume numbers, and each being listed as a publication either of the House of Commons or the House of Lords. A citation to these Sessional Papers can be deceiving, since some volumes are made up of separate papers paged individually and arranged either chronologically by day or alphabetically by primary subject. Cite the specific document by its title, with pertinent numbered sections or paragraphs (if the document is long), and page numbers. The volumes include well-arranged tables of contents and are indexed annually (see also 12.26).

N   1. House of Commons, "Present and Future Role of the Assistant Chief Education Officer," *Sessional Papers, 1982-83, Prison Education,* 25 April 1983, vol. 2, par. 9.14, p. 102.

B   United Kingdom. House of Commons. "Present and Future Role of the Assistant Chief Education Officer." *Sessional Papers, 1982-83, Prison Education,* 25 April 1983. Vol. 2.

PR   (United Kingdom. House of Commons 1983, vol. 2, par. 9.14, p. 102)

RL   United Kingdom. House of Commons. 1983. Present and future role of the assistant chief education officer. *Sessional Papers, 1982-83, prison education.* 25 April. Vol. 2.

PARLIAMENTARY DEBATES

12.28   Since 1909 the *Parliamentary Debates* have been published separately for the two houses. The name *Hansard* (for an original printer of the debates) often does not appear on the title pages of volumes issued since 1909, but it still has official sanction, and the debates are commonly referred to as *Hansard* or *Hansard's,* even though they are now published by HMSO (see 12.24). Use the title as it appears in the volume being cited. Series and volume numbers should also be cited:

N   [1]*Parliamentary Debates,* Lords, 5th ser., vol. 13 (1893), col. 1273.

B   United Kingdom. *Parliamentary Debates,* Lords. 5th ser., vol. 13 (1893), col. 1273.

PR   (United Kingdom 1893)

RL   United Kingdom. 1893. *Parliamentary Debates,* Lords, 5th ser., vol. 13, col. 1273.

N   [2]*Hansard Parliamentary Debates,* 3d ser., vol. 249 (1879), cols. 611-27.

B   United Kingdom. *Hansard Parliamentary Debates.* 3d ser., vol. 249 (1879), cols. 611-27.

PR   (United Kingdom 1879)

RL   United Kingdom. 1879. *Hansard Parliamentary Debates*. 3d ser., vol. 249, cols. 611-27.

Specific items in the *Debates* may be cited as follows:

N   [3]Winston Churchill, Speech to the House of Commons, 18 January 1945, *Parliamentary Debates,* Commons, 5th ser., vol. 407 (1944-45), cols. 425-46.

B   Churchill, Winston. Speech to the House of Commons, 18 January 1945. *Parliamentary Debates,* Commons, 5th ser., vol. 407 (1944-45), cols. 425-26.

PR   (Churchill 1945)

RL   Churchill, Winston. 1945. Speech to the House of Commons, 18 January. *Parliamentary Debates,* Commons, 5th ser., vol. 407 (1944-45), cols. 425-46.

BRITISH FOREIGN AND STATE PAPERS

12.29   The *British Foreign and State Papers* are arranged within the volumes alphabetically by country and, further, by subject:

N   1. Foreign Office, "Austria: Proclamation of the Emperor Annulling the Constitution of 4th March, 1849," *British Foreign and State Papers, 1952-53,* 41:1298-99.

B   United Kingdom. Foreign Office. "Austria: Proclamation of the Emperor Annulling the Constitution of 4th March, 1849." *British Foreign and State Papers, 1952-53.*

PR   (United Kingdom. Foreign Office 1952-53, 41:1298-99)

RL   United Kingdom. Foreign Office. 1952-53. Austria: Proclamation of the emperor annulling the constitution of 4th March, 1849. *British Foreign and State Papers, 1952-53.*

12.30   Reports are issued in pamphlet form by ministries, commissions, committees, and the like:

N   [1]Office of the Minister of Science, Committee on Management and Control of Research, *Report*, 1961, 58.

B   United Kingdom. Office of the Minister of

          Science. Committee on Management and
          Control of Research. *Report,* 1961.

PR   (United Kingdom. Office of the Minister of
          Science 1961, 58)

RL   United Kingdom. Office of the Minister of
          Science. 1961. Committee on Management and
          Control of Research. *Report.*

12.31 The early records titled *Calendar of . . .* are arranged chronologically. In some, numbered items—grants, leases, warrants,
pardons, and so on—appear within a "calendar" of no uniform duration. Dates therefore are essential in identifying the
items, although parenthetical references should be used for
these works only when reference lists include adequate cross-
references and when as much information as possible is given
in the text.

N   1. Public Record Office, "Queen Mother to
          Queen," 18 February 1581, *Calendar of State
          Papers, Foreign Series, of the Reign of
          Elizabeth [I]* (January 1581-April 1582)
          (London, 1907), nos. 58, 63.

B   United Kingdom. Public Record Office. "Queen
          Mother to Queen," 18 February 1581.
          *Calendar of State Papers, Foreign Series,
          of the Reign of Elizabeth [I]* (January
          1581-April 1582). London, 1907.

PR   (United Kingdom. Public Record Office 1907,
          nos. 58, 63)

RL   United Kingdom. Public Record Office. 1907.
          Queen Mother to Queen, 18 February 1581.
          *Calendar of State Papers, Foreign Series,
          of the Reign of Elizabeth [I]* (January
          1581-April 1582). London.

CANADIAN PUBLIC DOCUMENTS

12.32 Canadian government documents are issued by both houses of
the Canadian Parliament (Senate and House of Commons)
and by the various executive departments. Statutes are published in the *Statutes of Canada* and identified by calendar year
and by chapter (c.) number.

N   [1]House of Commons, *Order Paper and
          Notices,* 16 February 1972, 6.

B   Canada. House of Commons. *Order Paper and
          Notices,* 16 February 1972.

```
PR      (Canada 1972, 6)

RL      Canada. House of Commons. 1972. Order paper and
           notices, 16 February.

N          ²Statutes of Canada, 1919, 10 Geo. 5, c.
        17.

B       Canada. Statutes of Canada. 1919. 10 Geo. 5, c.
           17.

PR      (Canada 1919)

RL      Canada. 1919. Statutes of Canada. 10 Geo. 5, c.
           17.
```

Unpublished records are housed in the Public Archives of Canada (PAC) and identified by the name of the record group, series, and volume.

```
N          ³Public Archives of Canada, Privy Council
        Office Records, ser. 1, 1477: 147-49.

B       Canada. Public Archives of Canada. Privy
           Council Office Records. Ser. 1, vol. 1477.

PR      (Canada n.d.)

RL      Canada. Public Archives of Canada. Privy
           Council Office Records. n.d. Ser. 1, vol.
           1477.
```

DOCUMENTS OF INTERNATIONAL BODIES

12.33 Citations to publications and documents of international bodies such as the League of Nations and the United Nations (sometimes abbreviated UN, with no periods), should give the following information, more or less in the order shown, whenever it is available: authorizing body, topic or title, series number, place of publication, date, publication number, and page reference when applicable:

```
N          1. League of Nations, Monetary and
        Economic Conference: Draft Annotated Agenda
        Submitted by the Preparatory Commission of
        Experts, II, Economic and Financial, 1933,
        II.Spec.I.

B       League of Nations. Monetary and Economic
           Conference: Draft Annotated Agenda
           Submitted by the Preparatory Commission of
           Experts. II. Economic and Financial. 1933.
           II.Spec.I.
```

PR   (League of Nations 1933, II.Spec.I)

RL   League of Nations. 1933. *Monetary and economic conference: Draft annotated agenda submitted by the Preparatory Commission of Experts.* II. Economic and financial. II.Spec.I.

N   2. United Nations Secretariat, Department of Economic Affairs, *Methods of Financing Economic Development in Underdeveloped Countries,* 1951, II.B.2.

B   United Nations Secretariat. Department of Economic Affairs. *Methods of Financing Economic Development in Underdeveloped Countries.* 1951.

PR   (United Nations Secretariat 1951, II.B.2)

RL   United Nations Secretariat. Department of Economic Affairs. 1951. *Methods of financing economic development in underdeveloped countries.*

13 Preparing the Manuscript

Division of Responsibilities 13.1
Equipment 13.2
Entering Text 13.7
   Special Characters 13.8
   Stored Keystrokes 13.9
Editing Text 13.10
   Style Sheets 13.12
File Management 13.13
Backing up Files 13.14
Formatting Text 13.15
Entering Footnotes 13.17
Equations and Formulas 13.18
Tables 13.19
Computer Graphics 13.21
Printing 13.24
   Printer and Software Interface 13.25
   Special Features 13.26
   Typeface 13.27
   Resolution 13.28
   Speed 13.29
   Printing the Final Copy 13.30
Correcting and Erasing 13.31
   Correcting Typewritten Manuscripts 13.32
   Correcting Manuscripts to Be Photocopied 13.33
   Correcting Photocopies 13.34
Paper Stock 13.35
Duplicating 13.36

DIVISION OF RESPONSIBILITIES

13.1   The writer is responsible for the correct presentation of the entire paper—all the preliminary, illustrative, and reference matter as well as the text. The person preparing the manuscript, if other than the writer, is responsible for accurate transcription of the copy, the layout of the components as illustrated in chapter 14, and the general appearance of the final manuscript, but not for content.

EQUIPMENT

13.2   The options for preparing a manuscript will be limited by what equipment is available. When there is a choice of various typewriters, computer systems, or photocopiers to use in meeting the specifications set by the dissertation office or by a particular department or discipline, one must decide which to use. First, plan the form of the paper in as much detail as possible: the kind of notes needed, the special characters required, and the complexity of the format (e.g., equations, formulas, illustrations, tables, long footnotes, transcriptions, linguistic trees, computer graphics, music, and non-Latin alphabets). Second, become as familiar as possible with the potential and limits of each option (such as entering the manuscript on a computer system or typing it in its final form) to make sure the equipment being considered can produce the results desired. The suggestions given here pertain mainly to computer systems. Earlier editions of this manual give fuller instructions for preparing manuscripts on a typewriter.

13.3   For papers prepared on computer systems, select software *first;* then choose compatible hardware. Try to consult someone knowledgeable to make sure every piece of hardware will work with the software chosen.

13.4   Whenever possible, test samples of the kind of work to be done before making a commitment to use the proposed system. This step also makes one familiar with all the stages of the paper's development and with the computer's capabilities at each stage. For example, do not take it for granted that a particular printer will meet the specifications of a dissertation office for type resolution and the quality of photocopies made from its output. Be sure the dissertation secretary or thesis adviser approves the quality of the final printout, any duplicate copies, and the paper stock used.

13.5 The writer can best determine what equipment suits the paper's requirements. Certain guidelines that apply universally are discussed below.

13.6 Before preparing a paper on a computer system, become familiar with the information in its user's manual.

ENTERING TEXT

13.7 Usually the first step in producing a paper on a computer is to enter the text directly, using a standard keyboard. Text entry does not vary significantly from one system to another. The writer should be satisfied with the characteristics of the screen display—for example, resolution and background color—but the choice of these is somewhat subjective. It is also important that the computer system give the writer complete control over what portion of text is displayed on the screen and over positioning of the cursor. It should be easy to move the cursor anywhere in the text.

SPECIAL CHARACTERS

13.8 For papers that require special characters, computer systems offer a major advantage because they can often produce a far greater range than those that appear on the standard typewriter keyboard or even the most sophisticated electronic typewriters. Some systems let one use function keys or combinations of keys or special codes to enter diacritical marks, non-Latin characters, and math symbols. There are also systems that allow the "remapping" of standard keyboards (alternative keyboard functions) when text requires special characters. Such systems may display the alternative keyboard layout on the screen. Not all systems can display exactly the special characters that have been entered; sometimes they may be represented by combinations of standard characters. Some systems allow the creation of individual special characters and complete fonts.

STORED KEYSTROKES

13.9   If a paper includes a name, a term, or a phrase that will appear often, software that can "store" a sequence of keystrokes on a specific function key may speed text entry and improve accuracy. For example, instead of entering "University" many times in a paper, the individual keystrokes of this word could be "mapped" to a key that when hit once would enter the full word. Optimal word processing programs allow one to store libraries of such keystrokes. This function can be particularly useful for those using word processors that produce special characters as combinations of standard keyboard characters.

EDITING TEXT

13.10   For those who expect to revise a paper significantly or who simply want an efficient means of editing while entering the text, computer systems offer the advantage of modifying text quickly, easily, and accurately. Significant portions of a paper—entire paragraphs, a word misspelled throughout, and the like—can be revised, reformatted, and reprinted without rekeying correct portions and possibly introducing new errors. With most word processing systems it is possible to insert and delete text, move material from one location to another, replace sections with other sections, and automatically find text strings and replace them with other text strings.

13.11   To choose the right software for editing a paper, evaluate each package in terms of the writing assignment (especially any specifications that are unique) and editing preferences (e.g., composing at the terminal, significantly rewriting while entering, introducing notes early or late in the process). Though many systems have editing capabilities, individual software packages vary in power, speed, and flexibility. Certain software restricts some operations (for example, copying, moving) on large segments of the text; other software allows flexible management of segments of relatively unrestricted size. Most software packages include search and replace operations; more sophisticated packages include "wild card" routines, which match strings of any given prefix, suffix, or internal letter combination (e.g., *b*t* would match *bit, bat, bet,* etc.). The more powerful programs make changes based on various specified conditions (e.g., only in lines with a number, only in lines containing the letters *xyz*). Automatic hyphenation programs often divide words erroneously and should therefore be approached with great care. The safer and therefore recommended practice is to compose the material as *unjustified* text, that is, without end-of-line hyphenation and with ragged right-hand margins. Most word processing programs can eliminate *widows* and *orphans* (respectively, a paragraph-ending line appearing alone at the top of a page and the single opening line of a paragraph at the bottom of a page).

STYLE SHEETS

13.12 Many word processing systems have features that let the user format specific styles for repeated elements such as headings, subheads, paragraph indentions, lists, and block quotations. These styling features, sometimes called style sheets, eliminate the need to tailor these elements each time they come up, and writers are well advised to use them.

FILE MANAGEMENT

13.13 No matter what type of research paper is being processed, it is important to be able to manipulate files easily, to save and retrieve files, name and rename them, generate automatic backup copies, and delete and merge files. Long papers should be saved in several files; for example, one for each chapter (of about thirty pages). If the software generates lists, tables of contents, and other parts of the paper, it may be necessary to combine copies of the text files, save the composite file, and then process the paper as a whole. It is important to name files carefully in order to identify which generation of a particular component is being displayed on the screen or printed.

BACKING UP FILES

13.14 No matter what software or hardware is used, it is necessary to save copies of the work in progress. Preferably, both printouts and duplicate disks or tapes should be saved and dated so that there are always printed and electronic backups of every part of the paper at each stage of composition. Not doing so risks losing material that cannot be replaced.

FORMATTING TEXT

13.15   Formatting refers to positioning text for display, such as laying it out correctly for printing as specified in chapter 14. Some powerful formatting software can perform special functions, such as generating tables of contents and lists; managing headers and footers; controlling orphan lines; paginating; changing variable fields in the paper to text strings; producing computer graphics; positioning footnotes, tables, and illustrations at the appropriate places in the text and numbering them; and controlling the flow of text around such special components as equations, tables, and illustrations.

13.16   Page image formatting automatically positions text as it is being entered, usually for printing on an $8\frac{1}{2}$-by-11-inch page. The writer defines the page format by, for example, answering menu prompts or using a displayed ruler to set margins, page length, tab stops, and so on. Entry and formatting are nearly simultaneous, and the screen displays a full or partial view of the page almost as it would appear if printed. When the text being entered reaches the "end" of the page, a page break is automatically entered; as the text reaches the right margin, there is an automatic return to begin the next line. In unjustified text the right margin is uneven, or ragged, and there is no end-of-line hyphenation. When the justification feature is employed, hyphenation is automatically introduced when necessary at the end of the line, and the right margin is vertically aligned. Hyphenation features, however, are not always accurate, and this manual therefore recommends the unjustified format (see also 13.11, 14.3).

ENTERING FOOTNOTES

13.17   Those who are preparing a paper with footnotes should read the software documentation carefully before selecting the software and again before beginning to enter the text and notes. At the very least, a program should be able to place superscript numbers at the ends of referenced words and to single-space and double-space on the same page, so that notes at the bottom of the double-spaced text can be single-spaced, with a blank line between notes. Some sophisticated programs completely automate the process of arranging footnotes within the text, placing them on the proper pages and assigning them consecutive numbers. The more sophisticated the treatment of footnotes, the easier it will be to revise the paper, inserting new footnotes or rearranging them at each stage of composition. Of course, papers that rely instead on parenthetical references or endnotes can be revised more easily at any stage when using many standard word processing programs.

EQUATIONS AND FORMULAS

13.18 Only the most sophisticated word processing packages can produce anything more complex than simple linear equations. Usually it is necessary to create equations or formulas by using adjunct software. The task is made somewhat easier by following the guidelines of the American Mathematical Society's *Manual for Authors of Mathematical Papers,* which suggests ways of keeping equations simple (see the bibliography at the end of this manual). It may be necessary to treat equations and formulas as artwork (see 7.27–32).

TABLES

13.19 Some software packages offer the capabilities necessary to create tables, such as producing multiple tabs, making column adjustments, and performing spread-sheet management functions. Vertical as well as horizontal rules are often options, though these may also be added by hand (see chapter 6 for instructions on compiling tables and ruling them). Some powerful programs position tables within the text near references to them; position tables correctly on individual pages; automatically number the tables and adjust the numbering throughout revisions, including table numbers used in cross-references; and generate a list of tables for the preliminaries. Footnotes for tables, however, usually must be entered at the keyboard rather than generated and placed with tables automatically.

13.20   Some word processing programs automatically adjust cross-references when numbered elements of a paper (such as footnotes, equations, tables, and illustrations) are added or deleted.

COMPUTER GRAPHICS

13.21   If a paper includes bar graphs, line graphs, and pie charts, it may be advantageous to produce them with computer software. Computers can also be used to create and manipulate line drawings. Graphics drawn by a computer are usually vector graphics, which are created from coordinate points that can be interpreted (connected to form images) by display devices, printers, and plotters.

13.22   Graphics that do not originate on a computer, such as photographs or handmade drawings, can be scanned into the machine with a device that transforms the image into a digital representation called a bit map. Software exists for transforming vector graphics into bit maps. Graphics can also be entered with special digital-input cameras.

13.23   Depending on the capabilities of the system, computer graphics can be merged with the text or inserted as illustrations (see chapter 7).

PRINTING

13.24   Printing is an important consideration in preparing the research paper with a computer system. Clearly ascertain all printing requirements and be sure the necessary capabilities are available. Take into account the printer's compatibility with software, printing speed, resolution, and its ability to print graphics, equations, and special characters. Only after these characteristics have been tested should the manuscript be entered on a computer system.

PRINTER AND SOFTWARE INTERFACE

13.25   Among the most important considerations are the interfaces that link the word processing program to the printer. For example, there are two major types of ports (parallel and serial), and individual cable configurations vary. Software support for a printer should receive special attention, since not all software programs support all printers. Software should be able to adjust the mode of signals sent to the printer and to alter individual signals. Printers should be designed to allow easy control such as adjusting the interface signals using front panel controls instead of internal switches. The system used should be able to print only a part of the paper (e.g., one page with a revision on it), to print while editing (it can take several hours for some printers to print a paper), and to pause while printing (to change paper or daisy wheels or to clear jams).

Special Features

13.26   The formatted version of a paper prepared on a computer system should have only those characteristics that the printer can reproduce. For example, daisy wheel printers do not print italics as readily as they underline or print boldface characters. In choosing a printer, consider how the following features apply to the specific needs of the paper: underlining, using boldface or italics, shadowing, superscripting, typing special characters, variable feeding, color printing, providing variable type styles and pitch, and producing computer graphics. Other special features have to do with spacing between characters, words, and lines.

Typeface

13.27   Ornamental typefaces, including script, should never be used for term papers, theses, or dissertations. The eminently readable Times Roman is perhaps the best choice. Courier, which is much like a typewriter font, is also generally acceptable, but ask the department or the dissertation secretary about any special requirements. Type fonts that include italic are preferable. Either italics or underlining should be used throughout the paper, and no text should ever be both italicized and underlined. All type, including superscript numbers and letters, must be large enough and dark enough to be clearly legible even on microfilm. Twelve-point type (ten characters per inch) for text and ten-point (twelve characters per inch) for notes will meet the requirements of most institutions, but check with the dissertation office.

RESOLUTION

13.28 All theses and dissertations must meet the requirements of the degree-granting institution. Most will accept only papers printed on letter-quality daisy wheel or laser printers; but dot matrix printers, which are often faster and less expensive to operate, may be used for working drafts of a paper and of graphics. Dot matrix printers frequently feature three modes: draft, medium resolution, and "near letter quality." But "near letter quality" in this context is not what most advisers and dissertation secretaries mean when they specify a letter-quality printout. They usually mean the manuscript must be printed by a daisy wheel or laser printer on acid-free paper. Even very high resolution dot matrix printing is usually unacceptable. The final copy must be on acid-free stock or must photocopy well on such paper.

SPEED

13.29 Speed can be a major consideration in choosing a printer, since they vary in the number of characters per second (cps) they can type (e.g., 12–18, 25–35, 36–60, 80–120, 200 cps). Dot matrix printers are sometimes faster than daisy wheel or laser printers, but they offer the lowest resolution and do not satisfy many of the criteria listed in 13.26. Note that the rated speeds for printers, sometimes cited in the accompanying literature, may reflect optimum conditions. It is advisable, before selecting a printer, to determine how long it would take to print a paper of a given length, so as to anticipate how much time might be needed for printing drafts.

PRINTING THE FINAL COPY

13.30 Although drafts may be printed on pin-fed paper, dissertation offices usually require cut sheets or form-fed paper that will not leave ragged edges when separated. When using cut stock to print a long research paper, it may be best to use a sheet feeder. If photocopies are acceptable, it is sometimes more economical to print only one copy of the final version and then photocopy it onto acid-free paper.

CORRECTING AND ERASING

13.31   All corrections and erasures must be invisible. Since manuscripts of theses and dissertations generally must be typed or printed out, or else photocopied, on acid-free paper, several kinds of corrections are permissible.

CORRECTING TYPEWRITTEN MANUSCRIPTS

13.32   Correction papers, correction fluids, or self-correcting typewriter ribbons are acceptable if the coverage is complete. Deleting or inserting more than one character should be done by retyping. Many typewriters have a half-spacing function for adding missing characters. Whenever possible, such corrections should be made before the paper is removed from the typewriter.

CORRECTING MANUSCRIPTS TO BE PHOTOCOPIED

13.33   All the methods mentioned in 13.32 apply, in addition to using white correcting tape to cover lines and join portions of pages, since this tape does not show up on many photocopies. Manuscripts with extensive revisions of this kind may have to be fed into the photocopier one page at a time. Acid-free paper does not flow as smoothly through automatic feeders as lower-quality stock, which may be used for drafts to be reproduced this way, with the final version copied on acid-free paper.

CORRECTING PHOTOCOPIES

13.34   To cover specks or unwanted characters in a line that would otherwise not have to be retyped, use correcting fluid designed especially for photocopies.

PAPER STOCK

13.35 Whether a paper is typewritten or entered on a computer system, it should reach its final form as a correctly formatted text on the paper stock specified by the degree-granting institution. In the absence of such a directive, for archival purposes the American Library Association has established guidelines that recommend the use of acid-free paper—20-pound weight, neutral-pH paper that is labeled either "buffered" or as having a minimum 2 percent alkaline reserve. Photocopies should also be made on this type of paper. Some but not all stock referred to as "dissertation bond" meets these requirements. The normal page dimensions are $8\frac{1}{2}$ by 11 inches.

DUPLICATING

13.36 In using photocopiers to duplicate manuscripts, remember the following points: (1) ask to have the machine cleaned and toner checked before the paper is copied; (2) use only acid-free paper that has not been removed from the package until immediately before use, since the moisture in long-opened paper can create feeding problems; (3) when copying from acid-free paper to acid-free paper, feed the pages one by one; (4) if the stock is photocopy paper or somewhat lighter weight typewriting paper, feed it into large photocopiers fifty pages or fewer at a time; (5) check every copy to be sure that all are uniform and that no pages are missing; and (6) check for distortions in artwork, such as those caused by the 2 percent enlargement created by each photocopy generation.

14 Formats and Sample Layouts

Laying out the Text 14.2
  Margins 14.2
  Indention 14.4
  Spacing 14.5
  Pagination 14.6
Chapter Heads and Other Major Headings 14.10
  Subheads 14.11
  Laying out Footnotes on the Page 14.13
    Spacing, Indention, and Placement of
      Footnote Numbers 14.13
    Footnotes on a Short Page 14.15
    Footnotes in a Quotation 14.16
Sample Pages 14.18
  Title Page 14.18
  Table of Contents 14.19
    First Page of Contents 14.19
    Last Page of Contents 14.20
  List of Illustrations 14.21
  List of Tables 14.22
  Figure Set into the Text 14.23
  Broadside Figure 14.24
  Table without Rules 14.25
  Table with Horizontal and Vertical Rules 14.26
  Table with Spanner Heads and Blank Cells 14.27
  Table with Decked Heads 14.28
  Table with Note 14.29
  Broadside Table with Notes 14.30
  Table Set into the Text 14.31
  List of Abbreviations 14.32
  Glossary 14.33
  First Page of a Chapter 14.34

Text with Footnotes 14.35
Text with Footnotes Running to the Next Page 14.36
Text with Block Quotations of Prose and Poetry 14.37
Endnotes 14.38
Reference List 14.39
Reference List with Many Works by One Author 14.40
Bibliography with Works by the Same Author
   Arranged Chronologically 14.41
Bibliography with Works by the Same Author
   Arranged Alphabetically 14.42

14.1 This chapter offers suggestions, recommendations, and examples for formatting the term paper, thesis, or dissertation. It is intended not as an inflexible prescription, but as a guide and stimulus to the writer's own judgment. Special formatting requirements may indeed be mandated by some degree-granting institutions or academic departments, however, and they should be determined at the start. Once a suitable format has been decided on, the computer system's style sheet (see 13.12) will apply it consistently.

LAYING OUT THE TEXT

MARGINS

14.2 The normal page dimensions are 8½ by 11 inches. Leave a margin of at least one inch on all four edges of the page. Some institutions require more, particularly on the left, where binding reduces the margin.

14.3 Right margins should be justified (aligned) only if it can be done without leaving large gaps between words. When lines are automatically justified by a computer, all hyphenation must be carefully checked and adjusted (see 3.35–53, 13.16).

INDENTION

14.4 The critical rule for paragraph indention is consistency. Whether the amount is five or eight spaces or some other measure, it must always be the same. Word processing programs generally have a standard indention key. Block quotations (extracts) of prose should all be indented the same distance from the left margin of the text, and paragraph openings within them should have a consistent additional indention. Poetry treated as a block quotation may be indented a standard amount on the left, or the longest line may be centered on the full width of the text, so long as the choice is followed consistently for each extract.

SPACING

14.5   The text should be double-spaced except for block quotations, notes, captions, and long headings, which should be single-spaced with a blank line between items. This means that any computer system suitable for preparing research papers must be capable of double-spacing and single-spacing on the same page.

PAGINATION

14.6   Every page of the paper, including blank pages, must be assigned a page number. Although counted in the pagination, the number should not appear on the title page or on other display pages such as the copyright, dedication, epigraph, or part titles (see also chapter 1).

14.7   Number preliminary pages with lowercase roman numerals (v, vi, etc.) centered at the foot of the page, at least three-fourths of an inch from the bottom edge. The title page counts as page i.

14.8   Number the remaining parts of the paper, including text, illustrations, appendix, notes, and bibliography or reference list, with arabic numerals centered or flush right at the top of the page at a regular distance (e.g., three-fourths of an inch) below the top edge. On pages with major headings, however (such as the first page of a chapter or the bibliography), place the number at the foot of the page, centered at least three-fourths of an inch from the bottom edge. The pagination of the body of the paper begins with arabic 1 and runs consecutively to the end.

14.9   Alternatively, number all pages of the text and reference matter in the upper right corner, except pages with major headings (see 14.8), where the numbers should be centered below the text.

CHAPTER HEADS AND OTHER MAJOR HEADINGS

14.10   Headings for major sections of the paper (such as INTRODUC-TION, CHAPTER 1, BIBLIOGRAPHY) usually begin two inches from the top of the paper, often centered and typed in full capitals. Arabic numerals are recommended for chapter numbers, but roman numerals or spelled-out numbers may also be used as long as the choice is followed consistently. The chapter title, in the same style as the chapter number, follows after a blank line. Long chapter titles may need to be set in two or more lines, single-spaced, all centered or flush left, following the style chosen. No punctuation should be used at the ends. The text, whether for a chapter or for any other major section, should begin a regular distance below the last line of the heading. For style of chapter headings, see 1.36.

SUBHEADS

14.11   A *centered subhead* of more than forty-eight characters should be divided into two or more single-spaced lines, arranged in an inverted pyramid. A *sidehead* of more than half a line should be divided more or less evenly into two or more single-spaced lines, with runovers beginning at the margin. *Run-in paragraph headings* should be italicized or underlined and followed by a period. With all other subheads, omit punctuation at the ends of lines. For style and capitalization of subheads, see 1.37–38.

14.12   All subheads begin on the third line below the preceding text. If two or more subheads appear together without intervening text, leave a blank line between them. Also leave a blank line between the subhead and the text following. A page must never end with a subhead.

LAYING OUT FOOTNOTES ON THE PAGE

SPACING, INDENTION, AND PLACEMENT OF FOOTNOTE NUMBERS

14.13   Footnotes must be placed, or at least must begin, on the page where they are referred to. The text and footnotes are separated by a short rule, or *separator*. If a footnote runs over to the following page, a *continuation separator* should be inserted on that page. Each footnote must begin on a new line, indented the same amount as paragraphs in the text. Footnotes are usually single-spaced, with a blank line between notes.

14.14 Either of two styles may be followed in numbering footnotes. The simpler one is to use numerals on the line, followed by a period, as in the first example. The older style is to use superscript numerals like footnote numbers in the text, without punctuation. (Both styles are illustrated throughout this manual; see also 8.10.)

> 2. Marcel, *The Mystery of Being,* 1:42.
>
> [2]Marcel, *The Mystery of Being,* 1:42.

FOOTNOTES ON A SHORT PAGE

14.15 When the ending of a chapter does not fill a whole page, any footnotes that apply to that page should be arranged in the usual style after the separating rule immediately following the text rather than at the bottom of the page.

FOOTNOTES IN A QUOTATION

14.16 When a block quotation (5.30–34) includes one or more note references that form part of the extract, the corresponding footnotes should be placed beneath the quotation, separated from the last line by an eight-space rule (striking the underscore key eight times). The reference indexes and the footnotes should follow exactly the form used in the original (8.5). Note references added by the writer of the paper should be numbered in sequence with the paper's notes, with the footnotes placed at the bottom of the page.

14.17 Some word processing software can automatically number footnotes, place them on the correct pages, and adjust the spacing of text around them. For information on footnote citations with computer systems, see 13.17.

SAMPLE PAGES

14.18 All the information shown on this sample title page for theses and dissertations must be included. (For an explanation of the copyright page, which sometimes follows the title page, see 1.8.)

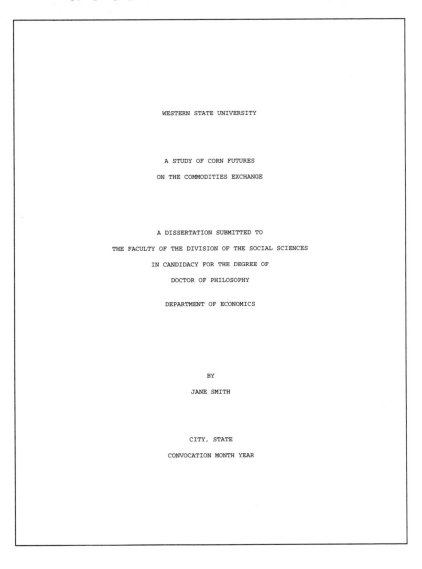

WESTERN STATE UNIVERSITY

A STUDY OF CORN FUTURES

ON THE COMMODITIES EXCHANGE

A DISSERTATION SUBMITTED TO

THE FACULTY OF THE DIVISION OF THE SOCIAL SCIENCES

IN CANDIDACY FOR THE DEGREE OF

DOCTOR OF PHILOSOPHY

DEPARTMENT OF ECONOMICS

BY

JANE SMITH

CITY, STATE

CONVOCATION MONTH YEAR

TABLE OF CONTENTS

FIRST PAGE OF CONTENTS

14.19 This example of the opening page of a table of contents includes part titles and one level of subhead.

CONTENTS

ACKNOWLEDGMENTS   vii

LIST OF ILLUSTRATIONS   viii

LIST OF ABBREVIATIONS   ix

Chapter

   1. INTRODUCTION   1

       Goals of the Study

               PART I. OVERVIEW

   2. POLICY DIVERGENCE AND TRADITIONAL RESEARCH   5

       Background of a Contrast: Divergence of Long-Term
         Care Outputs in Rural and Industrial States

       The Contrast and Its Causes

       Traditional Studies and the Failure to Provide
         a Plausible Explanation

   3. METHODOLOGY, RESEARCH PARADIGMS, AND THE ANALYTIC
      FRAMEWORKS GOVERNING BASIC ASSUMPTIONS   20

       Rationale for the Research Method

       Empirical Data and Their Collection

       Data Analyses

       Two Analytic Models

       Basic Assumptions

       A Dynamic View of the State Health Delivery System

         PART II. THE RURAL CASE STUDY

   4. THE COST-RECOVERY PROCESS IN RURAL STATES   36

       Why Health Delivery Costs Rose during the 1980s

       Why Rural States Needed to Act

       How Recipients of Health Care in Rural States
        Were Compensated

v

257

14.20 The sample below illustrates a style for the final page of a table of contents. It includes part titles and two levels of subheads.

PART TWO
THE DATA

Chapter   Page

9. DATA PRESENTATION.   83

10. ENERGY DIFFERENCES   94

11. ASPECTS OF NUCLEOSYNTHESIS WHERE PRECISE CAPTURE
    CROSS SECTIONS ARE REQUIRED   110

        Local Approximations   112

            Distortions.   115

            Deviation Ranges   118

        Process Branchings   120

        Abundance Characteristics Caused by a Pulsed
        Process with Time-Dependent Neutron
        Density and Temperature   124

            Radioactive Cosmic Clocks   135

12. SYSTEMATIC UNCERTAINTIES OF THE ACTIVATION
    TECHNIQUE   147

13. DETECTOR PROPERTIES AND THE RESULTS   179

14. AN ANALYSIS OF STELLAR NEUTRON CAPTURE RATES   200

15. CONCLUSIONS   234

Appendix

1. PLOTS OF THE DATA.   254

2. TABLES OF OBSERVED AND DERIVED PARAMETERS   260

REFERENCE LIST   267

vii

List of Illustrations

14.21 The following is a suggested format for a list of illustrations.

ILLUSTRATIONS

Figure   Page

1. Paul Gauguin, *Lutte de Jacob avec l'ange*, 1888   1

2. Jean Béraud, *The Church of Saint-Philippe-du-Roule*, 1877   7

3. Jean Baptiste Edouard Detaille, *En reconnaissance*, 1876   11

4. William Adolphe Bouguereau, *Bathers*, 1884   13

5. Jean Louis Ernest Meissonier, *Friedland, 1807*, 1875 . .   15

6. Henri Matisse, *Blue Still Life*, 1907   16

7. William Adolphe Bouguereau, *Youth of Bacchus* (sketch), 1884   21

8. Thomas Couture, *The Little Confectioner (Petit Gilles)*, ca. 1878   22

9. Alexandre Georges Henri Regnault, *Salomé*, 1870   23

10. Edouard Manet, *Portrait of Emile Zola*, 1868   28

11. Johan Barthold Jongkind, *The Church of Overschie*, 1866   43

12. Claude Lorrain, *The Ford*, 1636   44

13. Jean Baptiste Camille Corot, *View of Genoa*, 1834 . . .   48

14. Jean Baptiste Camille Corot, *Ville d'Avray*, ca. 1867-70   50

15. Claude Lorrain, *Landscape with the Voyage of Jacob*, 1677   54

16. Claude Monet, *Beach at Sainte-Adresse*, 1867 (Metropolitan Museum of Art).   69

17. Paul Cézanne, *View of Auvers*, ca. 1874.   77

18. Paul Cézanne, *Bathers*, ca. 1875-76   82

vi

LIST OF TABLES

14.22 The format for a list of tables is essentially the same as for a list of illustrations. See also 13.19–20.

TABLES

Table   Page

<table>
<tr><td>1.</td><td>Principal Ceramic Industries . . . .</td><td>4</td></tr>
<tr><td>2.</td><td>Ceramic Bodies and Their Characteristics . . . .</td><td>5</td></tr>
<tr><td>3.</td><td>Chronologial Sequence of Developments in Pottery and Ceramic Technology . . . .</td><td>7</td></tr>
<tr><td>4.</td><td>Relation between Pottery Making and Sedentism among Fifty-nine Societies . . . : . . . .</td><td>9</td></tr>
<tr><td>5.</td><td>Composition of the Earth's Crust . . . .</td><td>32</td></tr>
<tr><td>6.</td><td>Mineral Composition of Acid through Basic Rocks . . . .</td><td>34</td></tr>
<tr><td>7.</td><td>Properties of Some Clay Minerals . . . .</td><td>44</td></tr>
<tr><td>8.</td><td>Comparative Green Strength of Clays with and without Sand . . . .</td><td>70</td></tr>
<tr><td>9.</td><td>Temperature Conversion Chart, Celsius and Fahrenheit . . . .</td><td>83</td></tr>
<tr><td>10.</td><td>Pyrometric Cone Equivalent Temperatures . . . .</td><td>96</td></tr>
<tr><td>11.</td><td>Glaze Recipes . . . .</td><td>101</td></tr>
<tr><td>12.</td><td>Porosity of Some Fired Ceramic Products . . . .</td><td>116</td></tr>
<tr><td>13.</td><td>Postfire Coatings and Treatments for Pottery . . . . .</td><td>122</td></tr>
<tr><td>14.</td><td>Formulas for Calculating Volume of Geometric Shapes . . . .</td><td>130</td></tr>
</table>

ix

260

14.23 Note that extra space separates the figure (including its caption) from the text.

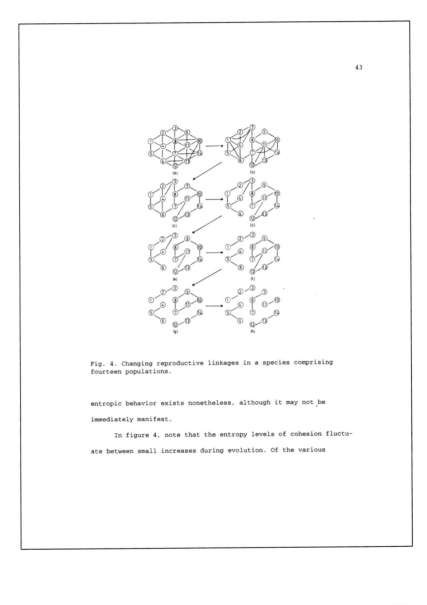

Fig. 4. Changing reproductive linkages in a species comprising fourteen populations.

entropic behavior exists nonetheless, although it may not be immediately manifest.

In figure 4, note that the entropy levels of cohesion fluctuate between small increases during evolution. Of the various

14.24 See chapter 7 for greater detail concerning illustrations in a paper and how to prepare them.

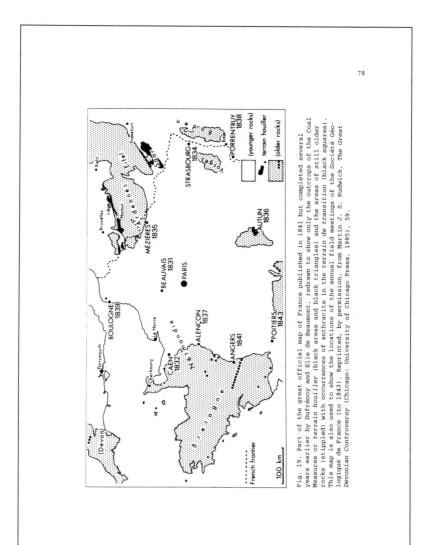

78

Fig. 19. Part of the great official map of France published in 1841 but completed several years earlier by Dufrénoy and Elie de Beaumont, redrawn to show only the outcrops of the Coal Measures or *terrain houiller* (black areas and black triangles) and the areas of still older rocks (stippled) with occurrences of anthracite in the *terrain de transition* (black squares). This map is also used to show the locations of the annual field meetings of the Société Géologique de France (to 1843). Reprinted, by permission, from Martin J. S. Rudwick, *The Great Devonian Controversy* (Chicago: University of Chicago Press, 1985), 59.

14.25

TABLE 7

MULTIPLE CORRELATION COEFFICIENTS
OF PROBABILITY FUNCTIONS

Range of Values	Number of Observed Values
0-.199	15
.2-.399	1
.4-.599	1

TABLE 8

CASES FILED, TERMINATED, AND PENDING IN THE COURT OF APPEALS
FOR THE THIRD CIRCUIT, FISCAL YEARS 1940-49, INCLUSIVE

Fiscal Year	Com- menced	Termi- nated	Pend- ing	Fiscal Year	Com- menced	Termi- nated	Pend- ing
1940	322	360	170	1945	299	268	226
1941	285	350	102	1946	197	274	149
1942	292	222	172	1947	266	216	199
1943	353	302	223	1948	287	250	236
1944	276	304	195	1949	128	113	251

TABLE 11

ESTIMATED NATIONAL INCOME OF INDIA, AT 1948-49 PRICES
1900-1901 TO 1950-51, BY SELECTED YEARS
(in Millions of Rupees)

	1900-1901	1910-11	1920-21	1930-31	1940-41	1950-51
Total income						
Amount	51,090	62,410	64,690	76,840	86,460	91,920
Index	100.0	122.1	126.6	150.4	169.2	179.9
Agricultural production						
Amount	39,760	44,330	38,070	45,980	45,340	44,050
Index	100.0	111.5	95.7	115.6	114.0	110.8
All other industries						
Amount	11,330	18,080	26,620	30,860	41,120	48,070
Index	100.0	159.6	234.9	272.4	362.9	424.8

Source: V. K. R. V. Rao, A. K. Ghosh, M. V. Divatia, and Um Datta, eds., *Papers on National Income and Allied Topics, Indian Conference on Research in National Income* (Bombay: Asia Publishing House, 1962) 2:22-23, table 3.

14.30 See 6.22. Note that when a table is placed broadside, its caption is at the binding and any notes are at the bottom of the table.

TABLE 12

VALUE ADDED BY MANUFACTURER PER PRODUCTION WORKER (IN DOLLARS), SOUTH BEND STANDARD METROPOLITAN AREA AND SEVEN SELECTED STANDARD METROPOLITAN AREAS, 1947

Census Group and Code Number	South Bend	South Bend Rank among Selected Standard Metropolitan Areas	Chicago	Indianapolis	St. Louis	Detroit	Toledo	Grand Rapids	Milwaukee
20. Food & related products	9,183	5	9,340	8,585	8,777	8,296	7,600	7,709	11,932
23. Apparel & related products	3,797	11	5,397	5,017	4,588	5,170	4,495	5,081	4,732
24. Lumber & related products, except furniture	5,629	2	5,503	3,700	4,464	7,569	5,124	5,168	5,262
26. Paper & related products	7,111	6	6,605	7,286	5,781	6,491	6,629	7,858	7,804
27. Printing & publishing industries	9,767	11	9,125	10,040	8,660	11,528	10,350	8,990	7,888
32. Stone, clay, & glass products	4,033	6	6,558	6,058	5,663	6,563	10,284	6,049	6,383
33. Primary metal industries	6,397	10	6,689	4,321	5,599	5,600	6,668	5,263	6,453
34. Fabricated metal products	5,351	4	6,534	5,037	5,687	5,569	5,759	5,884	6,928
35. Machinery, except electrical	6,048	10	6,656	5,502	5,756	6,847	7,298	7,022	6,368
36. Electrical machinery	6,613	6	6,682	6,614	6,054	6,862	5,823	. . .ᵃ	6,243
39. Miscellaneous manufactures	4,755	7	6,042	5,521	4,760	5,825	4,608	5,239	4,642

Source: U.S. Department of Commerce, Bureau of the Census, Census of Manufactures: 1947, vol. 3, Statistics by States (Washington, D.C.: Government Printing Office, 1948), 205-9, 308-18, 343-50, 479-81, 483, 648-49.

ᵃComplete figures are not provided by the Census.

124

TABLE SET INTO THE TEXT

14.31

45

"parapatric" by simply saying that sympatric speciation is an event

requiring no geographical component, whereas allopatric and parapatric

speciation have a geographical component.

Table 13. Four Classes of Linkage Pattern Changes When Information
Changes Are Great Enough to Disrupt or Prevent Cross-Linkages
between Phenotypes

	New pattern established and maintained	New pattern not established or maintained
Old pattern maintained	1. Immediate sympatric speciation	2. Stasis
Old pattern not maintained	3. Ecological sympatric speciation; parapatric speciation, allopatric speciation, or anagenesis	4. Extinction (local or species)

Speciation and Entropy Changes

One assumption implicit in the discussion of changes within

species was that changes in information were not of

the magnitude that would cause the population to become completely

disorganized. Complete disorganization may be manifested in two

ways, extinction and lineage splitting. The most radical change

that has been covered thus far is anagenesis, change without com-

plete disorganization. A species that avoids extinction and

becomes disorganized is a candidate for speciation. Speciation

LIST OF ABBREVIATIONS

14.32   See 1.27 and chapter 2.

ABBREVIATIONS

AM	*Annales des Mines*
ANH	*Annals of Natural History*
ASB	Académie des Sciences de Belgique
ASP	Académie des Sciences, Paris
Ath.	*Athenaeum* (newspaper)
BAAS	British Association for the Advancement of Science
BSGF	*Bulletin de la Société Géologique de France*
CPS	Cambridge Philosophical Society
CRAS	*Comptes-Rendus Hebdomadaires de l'Académie des Sciences* (Paris)
ENPJ	*Edinburgh New Philosophical Journal*
ER	*Edinburgh Review*
GDNA	Gesellschaft Deutscher Naturforscher und Ärzte
LG	*Literary Gazette*
MGS	*Memoirs of the Geological Survey of Great Britain*
n.d.	no date (on letter)
PGS	*Proceedings of the Geological Society of London*
PMJS	*Philosophical Magazine and Journal of Science*
pmk	postmark date (given only where manuscript does not provide day or month)
QR	*Quarterly Review*
RBAAS	*Reports of the British Association for the Advancement of Science*

GLOSSARY

14.33 See 1.28. The content of this example is taken, with some revisions, from the glossary in *Lithic Illustration: Drawing Flaked Stone Artifacts for Publication,* by Lucile R. Addington (Chicago: University of Chicago Press, © 1986 by the University of Chicago).

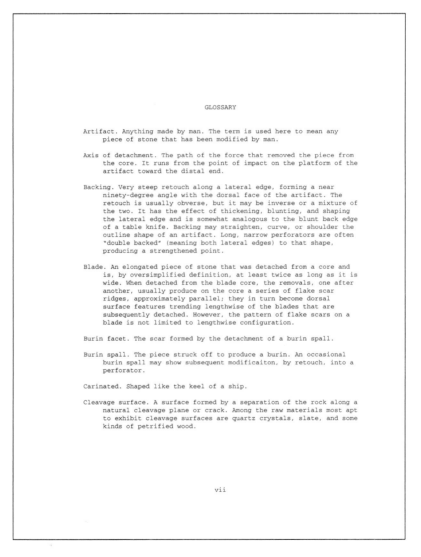

GLOSSARY

Artifact. Anything made by man. The term is used here to mean any piece of stone that has been modified by man.

Axis of detachment. The path of the force that removed the piece from the core. It runs from the point of impact on the platform of the artifact toward the distal end.

Backing. Very steep retouch along a lateral edge, forming a near ninety-degree angle with the dorsal face of the artifact. The retouch is usually obverse, but it may be inverse or a mixture of the two. It has the effect of thickening, blunting, and shaping the lateral edge and is somewhat analogous to the blunt back edge of a table knife. Backing may straighten, curve, or shoulder the outline shape of an artifact. Long, narrow perforators are often "double backed" (meaning both lateral edges) to that shape, producing a strengthened point.

Blade. An elongated piece of stone that was detached from a core and is, by oversimplified definition, at least twice as long as it is wide. When detached from the blade core, the removals, one after another, usually produce on the core a series of flake scar ridges, approximately parallel; they in turn become dorsal surface features trending lengthwise of the blades that are subsequently detached. However, the pattern of flake scars on a blade is not limited to lengthwise configuration.

Burin facet. The scar formed by the detachment of a burin spall.

Burin spall. The piece struck off to produce a burin. An occasional burin spall may show subsequent modificaiton, by retouch, into a perforator.

Carinated. Shaped like the keel of a ship.

Cleavage surface. A surface formed by a separation of the rock along a natural cleavage plane or crack. Among the raw materials most apt to exhibit cleavage surfaces are quartz crystals, slate, and some kinds of petrified wood.

vii

271

14.34 See also 13.18 for a discussion of producing special elements such as equations and formulas with computerized word processing.

CHAPTER 2

SPECIES, PHYLOGENETIC TREE TOPOLOGIES, AND ENTROPY

Different modes of speciation may predict different phylo-genetic tree topologies (Wiley 1981a, 2). For example, peripheral isolation results in the persistence of the ancestor (fig. 4.16a), whereas a large-scale geographical subdivision may cause ancestral extinction because neither descendant can be "identified" as the ancestor (rather, both "are") (fig. 4.16b). We may calculate the statistical entropy of each of these trees if we consider them to be directed graphs. In figure 4.16a, species X has one connection to itself (since it survives the speciation event) and one connection to Y, whereas Y has only a connection to X. The entropy of this tree, disregarding informational change, is

$$(2.1) \qquad H = -(2/3 \log_2 2/3) - (1/3 \log_2 1/3)$$
$$= 0.918 \, \text{bit}.$$

For figure 4.16b, X has connections with Y and Z and both Y and Z have connections only with X. The entropy is

$$(2.2) \qquad H = -(2/4 \log_2 2/4) - (2)(1/4 \log_2 1/4)$$
$$= 1.5 \, \text{bits}.$$

For figure 4.16c the situation is more complicated, because X is connected with itself twice and with Y and Z once for a total of four connections, whereas Y and Z are connected only to X. The

54

Text with Footnotes
14.35

theory for the examination of issues that Spencer had raised.
Where Spencer used economic terms still on the level of metaphor,
Lotka was able to construct in rudimentary form what was quite
literally an economy of nature.

The Economy of Nature

The search for an exact expression of these economic principles naturally led Lotka to the mathematical school of the
nineteenth-century economists represented by Augustin Cournot, Léon
Walras, Hermann Heinrich Gossen, and William Stanley Jevons.[59]
These were a school not in the sense of following the same program,
but in that they independently explored the use of mathematics in
economic analysis. It was to Jevons's *The Theory of Political
Economy* that Lotka turned for his principal model, adding a few
modifications culled from the early work of Vilfredo Pareto.[60]
Viewing economics as analogous to the physical sciences dealing
with statics and equilibrium, Jevons tried to develop a program of
scientific economics from Bentham's doctrine, creating out of the
combination a "calculus of pleasure and pain."[61]

Herbert Spencer, also following the utilitarian tradition, had
meanwhile framed the hedonistic principle in a psychological and

---

[59]C. Gide and C. Rist, *A History of Economic Doctrines,* 2d ed.
(London: George C. Harrap, 1948), 499-514.

[60]William Stanley Jevons, *The Theory of Political Economy,*
2d ed. rev. (London: Macmillan, 1879). Lotka used the 1911
edition, which has the same text. Also Vilfredo Pareto, *Manual of
Political Economy,* trans. A. S. Schwier (New York: Augustus M.
Kelley, 1971).

[61]Jevons, *Political Economy,* vii.

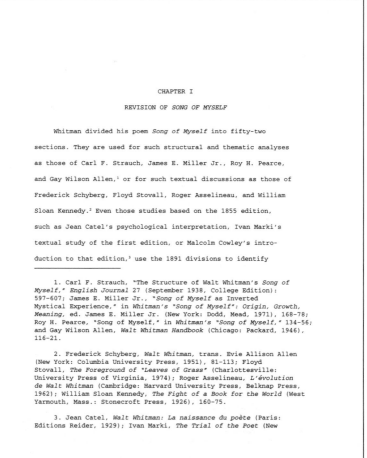

CHAPTER I

REVISION OF *SONG OF MYSELF*

Whitman divided his poem *Song of Myself* into fifty-two

sections. They are used for such structural and thematic analyses

as those of Carl F. Strauch, James E. Miller Jr., Roy H. Pearce,

and Gay Wilson Allen,[1] or for such textual discussions as those of

Frederick Schyberg, Floyd Stovall, Roger Asselineau, and William

Sloan Kennedy.[2] Even those studies based on the 1855 edition,

such as Jean Catel's psychological interpretation, Ivan Marki's

textual study of the first edition, or Malcolm Cowley's intro-

duction to that edition,[3] use the 1891 divisions to identify

---

1. Carl F. Strauch, "The Structure of Walt Whitman's *Song of
Myself*," *English Journal* 27 (September 1938, College Edition):
597-607; James E. Miller Jr., "*Song of Myself* as Inverted
Mystical Experience," in *Whitman's "Song of Myself": Origin, Growth,
Meaning,* ed. James E. Miller Jr. (New York: Dodd, Mead, 1971), 168-78;
Roy H. Pearce, "Song of Myself," in *Whitman's "Song of Myself,"* 134-56;
and Gay Wilson Allen, *Walt Whitman Handbook* (Chicago: Packard, 1946),
116-21.

2. Frederick Schyberg, *Walt Whitman,* trans. Evie Allison Allen
(New York: Columbia University Press, 1951), 81-113; Floyd
Stovall, *The Foreground of "Leaves of Grass"* (Charlottesville:
University Press of Virginia, 1974); Roger Asselineau, *L'évolution
de Walt Whitman* (Cambridge: Harvard University Press, Belknap Press,
1962); William Sloan Kennedy, *The Fight of a Book for the World* (West
Yarmouth, Mass.: Stonecroft Press, 1926), 160-75.

3. Jean Catel, *Walt Whitman: La naissance du poète* (Paris:
Editions Reider, 1929); Ivan Marki, *The Trial of the Poet* (New

1

passages that in the 1855 text were divided only by spaces between
line groups. Interpretations that strive to show Whitman's
reliance on Hindu texts, such as those of T. R. Rajasekhavaiah,
Som R. Raucham, and V. K. Chari,[4] use the numbering to indicate
lines while asserting that "the numerals division . . . scarcely
adds anything" to the poem.[5]

Analyses of technique compare the poem's structure to that
of a symphony,[6] an example of oratory,[7] the ocean,[8] and "a series
of spells evoking all the senses of man,"[9] each relying on the
fifty-two sections in order to identify passages. Discussions of
the formal poetics of *Song of Myself* focus on the resemblances of
Whitman's prosody to English translations of the Bible, on the
poem's language, on the rhetoric of the catalogs, on linguistic

---

York: Columbia University Press, 1976); Malcolm Cowley, ed.,
Complete Poetry and Prose of Walt Whitman (New York: Pellegrini
and Cudahy, 1948), 3-39.

4. T. R. Rajasekhavaiah, *The Roots of Whitman's Grass*
(Madison, N.J.: Farleigh Dickinson University Press, 1970), 386-
88; Som P. Raucham, *Walt Whitman and the Great Adventure with Self*
(Bombay: Manaktalas, 1967), 2-25; and V. K. Chari, *Whitman in the
Light of Vedantic Mysticism* (Lincoln: University of
Nebraska Press, 1964), 120-30.

5. Rajasekhavaiah, 386.

6. Basil de Selincourt, "The Form," in *Walt Whitman, a Critical
Study* (London: M. Secker, 1914), 94-115.

7. Schyberg, 241.

8. F. O. Matthiessen, "Only a Language Experiment," in
A Century of Whitman Criticism, ed. Edwin Haviland Miller (Bloomington:
Indiana University Press, 1969), 172-86.

9. Henry Seidel Canby, *Walt Whitman an American* (Boston:
Houghton Mifflin, 1943), 110.

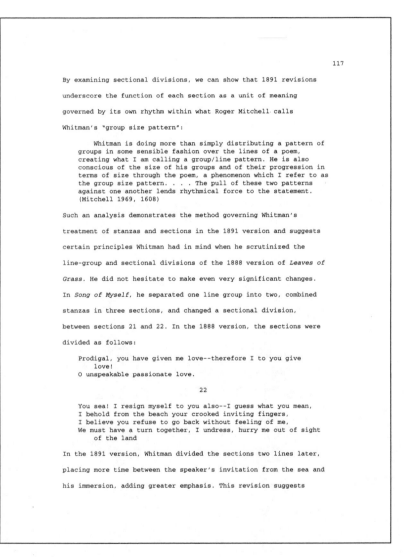

117

By examining sectional divisions, we can show that 1891 revisions

underscore the function of each section as a unit of meaning

governed by its own rhythm within what Roger Mitchell calls

Whitman's "group size pattern":

> Whitman is doing more than simply distributing a pattern of
> groups in some sensible fashion over the lines of a poem,
> creating what I am calling a group/line pattern. He is also
> conscious of the size of his groups and of their progression in
> terms of size through the poem, a phenomenon which I refer to as
> the group size pattern. . . . The pull of these two patterns
> against one another lends rhythmical force to the statement.
> (Mitchell 1969, 1608)

Such an analysis demonstrates the method governing Whitman's

treatment of stanzas and sections in the 1891 version and suggests

certain principles Whitman had in mind when he scrutinized the

line-group and sectional divisions of the 1888 version of *Leaves of*

Grass. He did not hesitate to make even very significant changes.

In *Song of Myself,* he separated one line group into two, combined

stanzas in three sections, and changed a sectional division,

between sections 21 and 22. In the 1888 version, the sections were

divided as follows:

> Prodigal, you have given me love--therefore I to you give
>   love!
> O unspeakable passionate love.

> 22

> You sea! I resign myself to you also--I guess what you mean,
> I behold from the beach your crooked inviting fingers,
> I believe you refuse to go back without feeling of me,
> We must have a turn together, I undress, hurry me out of sight
>   of the land

In the 1891 version, Whitman divided the sections two lines later,

placing more time between the speaker's invitation from the sea and

his immersion, adding greater emphasis. This revision suggests

14.38   See 8.2 for restrictions on the use of endnotes. This model, adapted from Wayne Booth's *Critical Understanding: The Powers and Limits of Pluralism* (Chicago: University of Chicago Press, © 1979 by the University of Chicago), shows content notes, the only endnotes recommended for use in papers, and then only with parenthetical references (see 10.19).

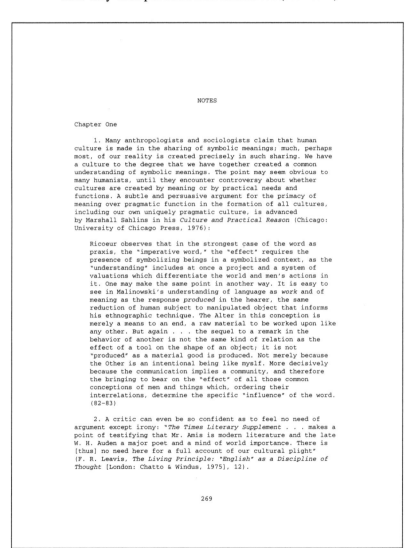

NOTES

Chapter One

1. Many anthropologists and sociologists claim that human culture is made in the sharing of symbolic meanings; much, perhaps most, of our reality is created precisely in such sharing. We have a culture to the degree that we have together created a common understanding of symbolic meanings. The point may seem obvious to many humanists, until they encounter controversy about whether cultures are created by meaning or by practical needs and functions. A subtle and persuasive argument for the primacy of meaning over pragmatic function in the formation of all cultures, including our own uniquely pragmatic culture, is advanced by Marshall Sahlins in his *Culture and Practical Reason* (Chicago: University of Chicago Press, 1976):

> Ricoeur observes that in the strongest case of the word as praxis, the "imperative word," the "effect" requires the presence of symbolizing beings in a symbolized context, as the "understanding" includes at once a project and a system of valuations which differentiate the world and men's actions in it. One may make the same point in another way. It is easy to see in Malinowski's understanding of language as *work* and of meaning as the response *produced* in the hearer, the same reduction of human subject to manipulated object that informs his ethnographic technique. The Alter in this conception is merely a means to an end, a raw material to be worked upon like any other. But again . . . the sequel to a remark in the behavior of another is not the same kind of relation as the effect of a tool on the shape of an object; it is not "produced" as a material good is produced. Not merely because the Other is an intentional being like myslf. More decisively because the communication implies a community, and therefore the bringing to bear on the "effect" of all those common conceptions of men and things which, ordering their interrelations, determine the specific "influence" of the word. (82–83)

2. A critic can even be so confident as to feel no need of argument except irony: "*The Times Literary Supplement* . . . makes a point of testifying that Mr. Amis is modern literature and the late W. H. Auden a major poet and a mind of world importance. There is [thus] no need here for a full account of our cultural plight" (F. R. Leavis, *The Living Principle: "English" as a Discipline of Thought* [London: Chatto & Windus, 1975], 12).

269

14.39 See 10.20–32. Note the use of initials for the first and second given names of authors, which is acceptable in a reference list when approved by the dissertation secretary or thesis adviser and followed consistently. Several works by one author are arranged here by date of publication, not alphabetically.

WORKS CITED

Abeloos, M. 1956. *Les métamorphoses.* Paris: Collection Armand Collin.

————. 1982. Development constraints in evolutionary processes. In *Evolution and development,* ed. J. T. Bonner, 313–32. New York: Springer-Verlag.

Blum, H. F. 1968. *Time's arrow and evolution.* 3d ed. Princeton: Princeton University Press.

Boucot, A. J. 1975. Standing diversity of fossil groups in successive intervals of geologic times viewed in the light of changing levels of provincialism. *Journal of Paleontology* 49:1105–11.

————. 1978. Community evolution and rates of cladogenesis. In *Evolutionary biology,* ed. M. K. Hecht, W. C. Steere, and B. Wallace, 11:545–655. New York: Plenum.

————. 1982. *Paleobiologic evidence of behavioral evolution and co-evolution.* Corvallis, Oreg.: by the author.

————. 1983. Does evolution take place in an ecological vacuum? *Journal of Paleontology* 37:1–30.

Bowler, P. J. 1983. *The eclipse of Darwinism.* Baltimore: Johns Hopkins University Press.

Brillouin, L. 1962. *Science and information theory.* New York: Academic Press.

Britten, R. J., and E. H. Davidson. 1969. Gene regulation for higher cells: A theory. *Science* 165:349–57.

Brooks, D. R. 1979. Testing the context and extent of host-parasite coevolution. *Sytematic Zoology* 29:192–203.

————. 1981a. Classifications as languages of empirical comparative biology. In *Advances in cladistics: Proceedings of the first meeting of the Willi Hennig Society,* ed. V. A. Funk and D. R. Brooks, 61–70. New York: New York Botanical Garden.

248

Reference List with Many Works by One Author

14.40 See 10.20–32. Note that in this format all works by the same author are arranged first by date, then alphabetically by title.

238

Thompson, W. R.
1923   La théorie mathématique de l'action des parasites entomophages. *Revue Générale des Sciences Pures et Appliquées* 34:202-10.

1929   On natural control. *Parasitology,* vol. 21.

1930a   *The biological control of insect and plant pests: A report on the organisation and progess of the work of Farnham House Laboratory.* London: King's Printer.

1930b   The principles of biological control. *Annals of Applied Botany* 17:306-38.

1930c   The utility of mathematical methods in relation to work on biological control. *Annals of Applied Biology* 17:641-48.

1937   *Science and common sense: An Aristotelian excursion.* London: Longmans, Green.

1939   Biological control and the theories of the interactions of populations. *Parasitology* 31:299-388.

1948   Can economic entomology be an exact science? *Canadian Entomologist* 80:49-55.

1956   The fundamental theory of natural and biological control. *Annual Review of Entomology* 1:379-402.

Varley, G. C.
1947   The natural control of population balance in the knapweed gall-fly. *Journal of Animal Ecology* 16: 139-86.

Verhulst, P.-F.
1838   Notice sur la loi que la population suit dans son accroissement. *Correspondances Mathématiques et Physiques* 10:113-21.

1845   Recherches mathématiques sur la loi d'accroissement de la population. *Nouveaux Mémoires de l'Académie Royale des Sciences et Belles-Lettres de Bruxelles* 18:3-38.

1847   Deuxième mémoire sur la loi d'accroissement de la population. *Mémoires de l'Académie Royale des Sciences des Lettres des Beaux-Arts de Belgique,* ser. 2, 20:3-32.

243

Rosecrance, Richard, ed. *The Dispersion of Nuclear Weapons
Strategy and Politics*. New York: Columbia University
Press, 1964.

_____. *Problems of Nuclear Proliferation*. UCLA Security
Studies Project no. 7. Los Angeles: University of
California, 1966.

Sabrosky, Alan. "The War-Time Reliability of Interstate
Alliances, 1816-1965." Paper delivered at the
Sixteenth Annual Conference of the International
Studies Association, Washington, D.C., 19-22 February
1975.

Sanders, Benjamin. *Safeguards against Nuclear
Proliferation*. Cambridge: MIT Press, 1975.

Savage, Leonard. *The Foundations of Statistics*. New York:
Dover, 1972.

Scheinman, Lawrence. *Atomic Energy Policy in France under
the Fourth Republic*. Princeton: Princeton University
Press, 1965.

Seshagiri, Narasimhiah. *The Bomb! Fallout of India's
Nuclear Explosion*. Delhi: Vikas, 1975.

Shapley, Deborah. "Nuclear Weapons History: Japan's Wartime
Bomb Project Revealed." *Science* 199 (13 January 1982):
152-57.

Singer, David, Stuart Bremer, and John Stuckey. "Capability
Distribution, Uncertainty, and Major Power War,
1820-1965." In *Peace, War and Numbers*, ed. Bruce
Russet, 193-206. Beverly Hills, Calif.: Sage, 1972.

Singer, David, and Melvin Small. *The Wages of War*. New
York: John Wiley, 1972.

Smith, H. "U.S. Assumes the Israelis Have A-Bomb or Its
Parts." *New York Times*, 18 July 1970.

Sommer, Theodore. "The Objective of Germany." *See* Buchan,
Alastair.

Stockholm International Peace Research Institute. *The Near-
Nuclear Countries and the NPT*. New York: Humanities
Press, 1972.

_____. *Nuclear Proliferation Problems*. Cambridge: MIT
Press, 1974.

Bibliography with Works by the Same Author Arranged Alphabetically

14.42

284

Downer, Alan S. "Prolegomenon to a Study of Elizabethan Acting."
Maske and Kothurn 10 (1965): 625-36.

Foakes, R. A. "The Players Passion: Some Notes on Elizabethan
Psychology and Acting." *Essays and Studies* 8 (1954): 62-77.

Greg, W. W. *Dramatic Documents from the Elizabethan Playhouses.*
2 vols. Oxford: Clarendon Press, 1931.

Harbage, Alfred. *Shakespeare and the Rival Traditions.* New York:
Macmillan, 1952.

————. *Shakespeare's Audience.* New York: Columbia University
Press, 1941.

Hillebrand, Harold Newcomb. *The Child Actors: A Chapter in
Elizabethan Stage History.* Urbana: University of
Illinois Press, 1926.

Hodges, C. Walter. *The Globe Restored.* London: E. Benn, 1953.

————. *Shakespeare and the Players.* London: E. Benn, 1948.

Hotson, Leslie. *Shakespeare's Wooden O.* London: Hart-David,
1959.

Isaacs, J. *Production and Stage Management at the Blackfriars
Theatre.* Shakespeare Association Pamphlet. London, 1933.

Joseph, B. L. *Elizabethan Acting.* 2d ed. London: Oxford
University Press, 1964.

King, T. J. "Staging of Plays at the Phoenix in Drury Lane, 1617-
42." *Theatre Notebook* 19 (1965): 1466-68.

Lawrence, W. J. *Old Theatre Days and Ways.* London: G. G. Harrap,
1935.

————. *The Physical Conditions of the Elizabethan Playhouses.*
Cambridge: Harvard University Press, 1927.

————. *Pre-Restoration Stage Studies.* Cambridge: Harvard
University Press, 1927.

Lithicum, M. Channing. *Costume in the Drama of Shakespeare and
His Contemporaries.* Oxford: Clarendon Press, 1936.

Nagler, A. M. *Shakespeare's Stage.* New Haven: Yale University
Press, 1958.

Selected Bibliography

GENERAL GUIDES

Baron, Dennis. *Grammar and Gender.* New Haven: Yale University Press, 1986.

Bernstein, Theodore M. *The Careful Writer: A Modern Guide to English Usage.* New York: Atheneum, 1977.

Booth, Wayne C., Gregory G. Colomb, and Joseph M. Williams. *The Craft of Research.* Chicago: University of Chicago Press, 1995.

The Chicago Manual of Style. 14th ed. Chicago: University of Chicago Press, 1993.

Fowler, H. W. *A Dictionary of Modern English Usage.* 2d ed. Revised by Ernest Gowers. Oxford: Clarendon Press, 1987.

Li, Xia, and Nancy B. Crane. *Electronic Styles: A Handbook for Citing Electronic Information.* 2d ed. Medford, N.J.: Information Today, 1996.

Miller, Casey, and Kate Swift. *The Handbook of Nonsexist Writing: For Writers, Editors, and Speakers.* 2d ed. New York: Harper and Row, 1988.

Monmonier, Mark. *Mapping It Out: Expository Cartography for the Humanities and Social Sciences.* Chicago: University of Chicago Press, 1993.

Perrin, Porter G. *Reference Handbook of Grammar and Usage.* New York: William Morrow, 1972.

Strunk, William, Jr., and E. B. White. *The Elements of Style.* 3d ed. New York: Macmillan, 1979.

Walker, Melissa. *Writing Research Papers: A Norton Guide.* 3d ed. New York: W. W. Norton, 1993.

Webster's New Biographical Dictionary. Springfield, Mass.: Merriam-Webster, 1983.

Webster's New Geographical Dictionary. Springfield, Mass.: Merriam-Webster, 1984.

Webster's Standard American Style Manual. Springfield, Mass.: Merriam-Webster, 1985.

Weidenborner, Stephen, and Domenick Caruso. *Writing Research Papers: A Guide to the Process.* 4th ed. New York: St. Martin's Press, 1994.

Williams, Joseph M. *Style: Toward Clarity and Grace.* Chicago: University of Chicago Press, 1990.

BIOLOGICAL SCIENCES

Council of Biology Editors Style Manual Committee. *Scientific Style and Format: The CBE Manual for Authors, Editors, and Publishers.* 6th ed. New York: Cambridge University Press, 1994.

Zweifel, Frances W. *A Handbook of Biological Illustration.* 2d ed. Chicago: University of Chicago Press, 1988.

ENGINEERING

American Institute of Chemical Engineers. *Guide for Writers and Speakers.* New York: American Institute of Chemical Engineers, 1978.

Institute of Electrical and Electronics Engineers. "Information for IEEE Authors." *IEEE Spectrum* 2 (August 1965): 11–15.

Kirkman, John. *Good Style: Writing for Science and Technology.* New York: Chapman and Hall, 1992.

Society of Mining Engineers. *Author's Guide.* Littleton, Colo.: Society of Mining Engineers/AIME, 1983.

GEOPHYSICAL SCIENCES

Cochran, Wendell, Peter Fenner, and Mary Hill, eds. *Geowriting: A Guide to Writing, Editing, and Printing in Earth Science.* Alexandria, Va.: American Geological Institute, 1984.

HUMANITIES

Achtert, Walter S., and Joseph Gibaldi. *The MLA Style Manual.* New York: Modern Language Association of America, 1985.

Gibaldi, Joseph. *MLA Handbook for Writers of Research Papers.* 4th ed. New York: Modern Language Association of America, 1995.

Hammond, N. G. L., and H. H. Scullard. *The Oxford Classical Dictionary.* 2d ed. New York: Oxford University Press, 1970.

LAW AND POLITICS

Garner, Diane L., and Diane H. Smith, eds. *The Complete Guide to Citing Government Information Resources: A Manual for Writers and Librarians,* rev. ed. (Bethesda, Md.: Congressional Information Service for the Government Documents Round Table, American Library Association, 1993).

Monthly Catalog of United States Government Publications. Washington, D.C.: Government Printing Office.

Morehead, Joe, Jr. *Introduction to United States Public Documents.* 3d ed. Littleton, Colo.: Libraries Unlimited, 1983.

———. *Essays on Public Documents and Government Policies.* Technical Services Quarterly series, vol. 3. Binghamton, N.Y.: Haworth, 1986.

Pemberton, John E. *The Bibliographic Control of Official Publications.* Elmsford, N.Y.: Pergamon, 1982.

Rodgers, Frank. *A Guide to British Government Documents.* New York: H. W. Wilson, 1980.

Schmeckebier, Laurence F., and Roy B. Eastin. *Government Publications and Their Use.* 2d ed. Washington, D.C.: Brookings Institution, 1969.

A Uniform System of Citation. 15th ed. Cambridge: Harvard Law Review Association, 1991.

United States Government Printing Office. *Style Manual.* Rev. ed. Washington, D.C.: Government Printing Office, 1984.

The University of Chicago Manual of Legal Citation. Edited by the staff of the *University of Chicago Law Review* and the University of Chicago Legal Forum. Rochester, N.Y.: Lawyers Co-operative Publishing Co., 1989.

MATHEMATICS

Higham, Nicholas J. *Handbook of Writing for the Mathematical Sciences.* Philadelphia: Society for Industrial and Applied Mathematics, 1993.

A Manual for Authors of Mathematical Papers. 8th ed. Providence, R.I.: American Mathematical Society, 1990.

Swanson, Ellen. *Mathematics into Type: Copyediting and Proofreading of Mathematics for Editorial Assistants and Authors.* Rev. ed. Providence, R.I.: American Mathematical Society, 1986.

PHYSICAL SCIENCES

Day, Robert A. *How to Write and Publish a Scientific Paper.* 4th ed. Phoenix, Ariz.: Oryx Press, 1994.

Dodd, Janet S., ed. *The ACS Style Guide: A Manual for Authors and Editors.* Washington, D.C.: American Chemical Society, 1986.

Hathwell, David, and A. W. Kenneth Metzner, eds. *Style Manual.* 3d ed. New York: American Institute of Physics, 1978.

Hopkins, Jeanne. *Glossary of Astronomy and Astrophysics.* 2d ed. Chicago: University of Chicago Press, 1980.

ISO (International Standards Organization). *General Principles concerning Quantities, Units, and Symbols.* ISO 31-0:1981. Geneva: International Standards Organization, 1981.

Katz, Michael J. *Elements of the Scientific Paper: A Step-by-Step Guide for Students and Professionals.* New Haven: Yale University Press, 1986.

SOCIAL SCIENCES

Becker, Howard S. *Writing for Social Scientists: How to Start and Finish Your Thesis, Book, or Article.* Chicago: University of Chicago Press, 1986.

Robert M. Emerson, Rachel I. Fretz, and Linda L. Shaw. *Writing Ethnographic Fieldnotes.* Chicago: University of Chicago Press, 1995.

Publication Manual of the American Psychological Association. 4th ed. Washington, D.C.: American Psychological Association, 1994.

Index

a, an. See articles (parts of speech)
abbreviations, 2.1–28
  A.D., 2.56
  address, forms of, 2.1, 2.3–10
  addresses, street, 2.15
  A.M., 2.57
  B.C. and B.C.E., 2.56
  in bibliographies, 2.12, 2.13
  capitalization, 2.11, 2.12, 2.24
  capital letters as, 3.50
  C.E., 2.56
  cf., 2.23, 2.26, 8.152
  civil titles, 2.7–8
  in classical references, 2.22, 8.119
  in column headings, 6.35, 6.48–49
  company names, 2.12
  constitutions and bylaws, 2.27
  countries, 2.13
  days and months, 2.55
  degrees, 2.5, 3.50
  Dr., 2.6
  ed., trans., comp., 2.26, 8.40, 10.31
  e.g., 2.23, 2.26, 3.78
  equations, 2.65
  eras, 2.56
  et al., 2.26, 10.6–8
  etc., 2.23, 2.26, 3.70
  f., ff., 8.71
  geographical names, 2.13–15
  ibid., 2.23, 2.26, 8.85–87
  id., 2.26, 8.86
  idem, 8.86, 8.87
  i.e., 2.23, 2.26, 3.78
  journal titles, 8.19
  keys to illustrations, 7.17
  law reviews, 2.27
  loc. cit., 8.84
  in mathematical text, 2.65
  measurements, 2.16–17
  military titles, 2.7–8

n.d., 2.26, 8.67, 10.25
  notes, 8.17–20
  n.p., 2.26, 8.55, 8.56
  op. cit., 8.84
  ordinal numbers, 2.30
  organizations, 2.11–12
  p., pp., 2.26, 8.70, 10.13
  parenthetical references, 2.12, 2.23
  parts of work, 2.18, 8.18
  periods, 2.2, 2.11, 3.6, 3.56, 3.103
  personal names, 2.2
  plurals, 2.26, 3.6
  P.M., 2.57
  professional titles, 2.3–10
  pseud., 8.28–29
  publishers, 8.57
  in reference lists, 10.30–31
  religious titles, 2.7–8
  Saint, 2.9–10, 2.14
  scholarly, 2.23, 2.26
  scholarly works, 2.18–23
  scientific usage, 2.64
  scripture, 2.20–21
  social and professional titles, 2.3–10
  Sr., Jr., III, and *IV,* 2.4
  state names, 2.13
  street and the like, 2.15
  s.v., 2.23, 2.26, 8.112
  in tables, 6.35, 6.48–49
  UN, 12.33
  unpublished manuscript types, 2.19
  USSR, 2.13
  v., vs., 2.26, 8.135
  weights and volumes, 2.16–17
  years, 2.52
  See also list of abbreviations
abstract, 1.13, 1.32
accents, 13.8
acid-free paper, 13.28, 13.33, 13.35, 13.36
accuracy of quotations, 5.3

Index

acknowledgments, 1.26
  for illustrations, 7.20
  in notes, 8.3
  preface containing, 1.25
  in table of contents, 1.13
A.D., 2.56
address, forms of, 2.1, 2.3–10
addresses, street. *See* street addresses
adhesives for mounting illustrations,
  7.39–42
adjectives
  capitalization of, 4.2–3
  centuries used as, 2.53
  comma separating, 3.80
  in compounds, 3.22–24, 3.27–33
  predicate, 3.23
adverbs
  in compounds, 3.22
  conjunctive, 3.76
  transitional, 3.86
aircraft, 4.26
alphabetizing
  anonymous works, 9.31
  Arabic names, 9.19
  articles in, 9.27, 9.31
  authors' names, 9.14–26
  bibliographies, 9.14–26
  Chinese names, 9.20
  compound names, 9.17
  family members, 9.23–24
  foreign names, 9.18–22
  glossaries, 1.28
  Japanese names, 9.21
  letter by letter, 9.15
  list of abbreviations, 1.27
  Mc, M, Mac, 9.15–16
  names with particles, 9.15
  person, place, thing, 9.32
  pseudonyms, 9.26
  references within note, 11.66
  religious names, 9.25
  Spanish names, 9.18
  Sr., Jr., III, IV, 9.24
  St., Saint, 9.15–16
  titles of works, 9.27, 9.31
  works by same author, 9.27–29, 10.21
A.M., 2.57
American Library Association paper standards, 13.35
ampersand (&), 8.59, 10.4
annotated bibliographies, 9.36
anonymous author, 8.30, 9.31
Apocrypha, 2.20–21, 4.21, 8.129
apostles, 2.9
apostrophe
  plurals of letters and abbreviations, 3.6

possessives, 3.7–11
appendix, 1.39–45
  illustrations in, 1.39, 7.4
  location, 1.40
  long quotations in, 5.14
  numbering, 1.41
  page numbers, 1.44, 14.8
  photocopied documents, 1.44
  references to, 4.13
  spacing, 1.43
  tables in, 1.39, 6.14, 8.4
  title, 1.42
  translations in, 4.33
arabic numerals
  chapter numbers, 1.17, 14.10
  collections of inscriptions, 8.126
  enumerations, 2.70–73
  figure numbers, 1.19, 7.13
  note numbers, 1.46, 8.7
  outlines, 2.73
  page numbers, 1.4, 14.8
  page references, 8.83
  parts of work, 2.44, 2.46, 8.83, 8.121
  scripture references, 2.20
  table numbers, 1.24, 6.13, 6.28
  volume numbers, 8.80, 8.101, 8.126
article, 2.27
articles (parts of speech)
  in alphabetizing, 9.27, 9.31
  capitalization, 4.6–7
  with newspapers, 8.110
  omission of, 8.95, 8.110
articles (periodical)
  artwork for, 7.27
  book reviews, 8.117, 11.46
  encyclopedias and dictionaries, 8.51,
    8.112, 11.42–43
  first, full reference, 8.22, 8.97–110
  journals, 8.99–103, 8.111, 10.25, 11.39–
    40
  magazines, 8.104, 8.111, 10.25, 11.41
  newspapers, 8.105–10, 8.111, 8.138,
    10.25, 11.44–45, 11.47
  old and new series, 8.102
  page references, 8.71–72
  quotation marks for titles, 4.17, 9.34,
    11.22, 11.28
  in reference lists, 10.29–30
  repeated references, 11.45
  subsequent references, 8.111
  titles within titles, 11.22–23
artwork. *See* illustrations
artworks, 8.147, 11.63–64
asterisk, for notes, 6.55–57
author-date system (parenthetical references), 10.2–19

author's name, 10.2–11, 10.18, 11.3–15
book title and subtitle, 10.26
constitutional citations, 12.21
cross-references, 8.150, 10.10, 10.22,
    11.2, 12.1
date of publication, 10.2, 10.11
manuscript collections, 10.16
newspapers, 10.25
notes with, 10.19
page references, 10.12–14
public documents, 12.2
See also parenthetical references; refer-
    ence list
author's name
alphabetizing, 9.14–26
anonymous work, 8.30
author-date system, 10.2–11, 10.18,
    11.3–15
in bibliographies, 8.42, 9.9–34, 11.3–15
classical works, 8.122
coauthors, 8.31–33, 8.89, 9.28–29, 10.4,
    10.6–8, 11.4–6
collected works, 11.13
complete work within another work,
    11.28
computer programs, 8.140
corporate body as, 8.35, 11.10
cross-references, 10.22, 11.2, 11.9
documentation systems compared,
    11.3–15
editor also named, 11.34
editor or compiler as, 8.36, 11.11
first, full reference, 8.26–36, 8.100
ibid., idem, 8.85, 8.86
initials, 8.26, 14.39
introduction, preface, or foreword,
    8.43, 11.24
multiauthor works, 8.31–33, 8.89, 9.28–
    29, 10.4, 10.6–8, 11.4–6
multiple works, 9.27–34
notes, 8.26–36, 8.40–43, 8.88–89, 8.115,
    8.122, 8.131, 8.140, 11.3–15
order of, 8.26, 8.31, 9.9–10, 9.21, 9.246
parenthetical references, 10.2–11,
    10.18, 11.3–15
part of work, 11.26–27
pseudonyms, 8.27–29, 9.26, 11.9
public documents, 11.32, 12.4
reference lists, 10.21, 10.24, 11.3–15
religious names, 9.25
reports, 11.32
shortened references, 8.88–89
in title of work, 8.42
title with, 8.34
translated or edited works, 11.12
unknown, 9.31, 11.7–8

unpublished works, 8.131
well-known authors, 8.115

back matter (reference matter), 1.39–47
glossary, 1.28–30
headings for, 1.39, 1.41, 1.46, 9.2,
    14.33, 14.39
pagination, 1.3–4, 1.44, 14.8
in table of contents, 1.13
See also appendix; bibliography; end-
    notes; reference list
B.C., 2.56
B.C.E., 2.56
Bible
abbreviations, 2.20–21
chapter and verse, 2.20–21, 2.46, 3.90,
    8.129
facts of publication, 8.51
fragments, 2.47
titles, 2.20–21, 4.21
versions, 2.21
bibliography, 9.1–36
abbreviations, 2.12–13
alphabetizing, 9.14–26, 9.32
annotated, 9.36
arrangement of, 9.3–6, 9.14–34
authors' names, 8.42, 9.9–34, 11.3–15
books, 11.3–38
capitalization, 4.5–12
chronological order, 9.3, 9.6
classification, 9.3–6
constitutions, 12.21
cross-references, 11.2
documentation systems compared, 9.7–
    13, 11.1–68
encyclopedia articles, 8.112, 11.42–43
headings, 9.2–6, 14.39
indention, 9.8
interviews, 11.48–50
manuscript collections, 4.20
microform editions, 11.51
multiauthor works, 9.28–29
music, 11.58–59
newspapers, 11.44–45
page numbers in, 9.12–13
pagination of, 14.8
performances, 11.62
periodicals, 11.39–41
pseudonyms, 9.26, 11.9
public documents, 12.1–33
punctuation, 3.90, 8.55, 8.57, 9.11
recordings, 11.60–61
reference books, 8.112, 11.42–43
reviews, 11.46–47
sample pages, 14.41, 14.42
spacing, 1.2, 9.8

bibliography (*continued*)
  subheads, 9.3–5
  titles of works, 4.5–13, 9.31, 9.34–35
  unpublished materials, 11.52–57
  works of art, 11.63–64
billion, 2.35, 2.42
blank page, 1.8, 1.11, 14.6
block quotations, 5.30–34
  beginning with new paragraph, 5.30
  capitalization of first word, 5.30
  computer programs for, 5.5
  defined, 5.4
  ellipsis points in, 5.33–34
  enumerations, 5.14
  headings and subheadings within, 5.15
  indention, 5.4, 5.30, 5.32, 14.4
  of letters, 5.13
  notes within, 8.5, 14.16
  outlines, 5.14
  parenthetical reference with, 5.30
  quotations within, 5.11
  with quoted fragments, 5.31
  sample page, 14.37
  spacing, 1.2, 5.4, 5.6, 14.5
boldface, 13.26
book, 2.18, 2.26, 3.20
book reviews, 8.117, 11.46
books, citation of
  author's name, 8.26–36, 11.3–15
  documentation systems compared,
    11.3–38
  edition, 4.18, 8.44–48, 8.124, 8.137–38,
    11.18–20, 11.51
  editor, translator, or compiler, 8.40–42
  facts of publication, 8.51–69
  first, full reference, 8.22–83
  foreign language, 11.25
  impression, 11.18
  introduction, preface, or foreword,
    11.24
  multivolume works, 8.74–83, 11.14–15
  note references, 8.23–96
  page references, 8.70–73
  parts of, 11.24, 11.26–28
  privately printed, 11.29–30
  proceedings, 11.34–36
  in reference lists, 10.26
  reference works, 8.51, 8.112, 11.42–43
  reports, 11.33–34, 11.36
  as secondary source of quotation, 11.31
  series, 4.15, 4.18, 8.49–50, 11.16–17
  short title, 8.93–96
  subsequent references, 8.20, 8.84–96
  title, 4.5–12, 4.16, 8.37–39, 8.93–96,
    9.34
  title within title, 11.21–23

works of art reproduced in, 11.64
  yearbooks, 11.37–38
brackets, 3.99–100
  with date of publication, 8.68, 11.54
  interpolations in quotations, 3.99,
    3.110, 5.35
  within parentheses, 3.99
  phonetic transcriptions, 3.100
  punctuation with, 3.105, 3.108, 3.110
British currency, 2.40–41, 3.51
British public documents, 12.22–31
broadside pages
  illustrations on, 7.9, 14.24
  tables on, 6.22, 14.30
bulletins, 4.16. *See also* public documents
bylaws, 2.27

ca., 2.26
Canadian public documents, 12.32
capitalization, 4.1–13
  abbreviations, 2.11, 2.12, 2.24
  in bibliographies, 4.5–13, 10.26–30
  book, chapter, 2.18
  chapter titles, 1.15, 1.36, 14.10
  foreign titles, 4.10–12, 8.210, 9.35,
    8.100, 10.30, 11.25
  headline-style, 1.23, 4.5–8, 6.27–28,
    6.38, 8.100, 10.27, 10.30, 14.21
  legends, 1.23, 7.14, 14.21
  list of illustrations, 1.23, 14.21
  list of tables, 1.24
  original, 4.8
  parts of work, 2.18, 4.13, 10.28
  periodical titles, 8.100, 10.30
  prepositions, 4.6–7
  proper adjectives, 4.2–3
  proper nouns, 4.1–3
  question within sentence, 3.60
  quotation, 5.26, 5.30
  in reference lists, 10.26–30
  section titles, 1.15–16
  sentence-style, 2.73, 4.5, 4.9, 6.27,
    6.38, 9.35, 10.26, 10.28–29,
    11.25
  series, 10.27
  subheads, 1.16
  subtitles, 4.6, 10.26, 11.25
  table of contents, 1.15–16
  tables, 1.24, 6.27–28, 6.38
  titles of works, 4.5–13, 8.100, 8.120,
    9.35, 10.26, 10.30, 11.25
capital letters, for abbreviations, 2.11, 3.5,
    3.6, 3.50
captions. *See* legends
case. *See* capitalization; capital letters
C.E., 2.56

cents, 2.40
centuries, 2.53
cf., 2.23, 2.26, 8.152
chapter, 2.18
chapter heads. *See* chapter titles
chapter numbers, 1.36
  arabic numerals for, 1.17, 14.10
  roman numerals for, 1.17
  style for, 14.10, 14.34
  in table of contents, 1.13, 1.17
  in text references, 2.18
chapters, 1.36
  citation of, 4.17, 8.25, 8.38, 8.93, 10.28,
    11.26–27
  note numbering, 1.46, 8.12
  sections, 1.37–38
  See also chapter numbers; chapter titles
chapter titles
  epigraphs with, 5.9
  style for, 1.13, 1.15, 1.34, 1.36, 14.10,
    14.34
  in table of contents, 1.13, 1.17
  See also chapter numbers; chapters
charts, 7.4, 7.30, 13.21
chemical terms, 3.25, 6.28
Chinese names, 9.20
chronological order, 9.3, 9.6
churches, 2.61
church fathers, 2.9
CIS/Index (*Congressional Information Ser-
    vice Index*), 12.7
citation
  books, 8.23–96, 11.3–38
  classical works, 2.22, 2.46–47, 8.51,
    8.119–27
  documentation systems compared,
    11.1–68
  encyclopedia articles, 8.51, 8.112,
    11.42–43
  foreign works, 9.35, 11.25
  interviews, 8.118, 11.48–50
  microform editions, 8.137–38, 11.51
  music, 8.142–43, 8.146, 11.47, 11.58–59
  newspapers, 8.105–11, 8.138, 11.44–45
  performances, 8.146, 11.47, 11.62
  periodical articles, 8.19, 8.99–103,
    8.111, 8.117, 11.39–41
  public documents, 12.1–33
  recordings, 8.144–45, 11.60–61
  reviews, 8.117, 11.46–47
  unpublished materials, 8.83, 8.130–32,
    11.52–57
  works of art, 8.147, 11.63–64
  See also bibliography; notes; parentheti-
    cal references; reference list
city. *See* place of publication

civil titles, 2.7–8
classical works, citation of, 8.119–27
  abbreviations, 2.22, 8.119
  author's name, 8.122
  facts of publication, 8.51, 8.123
  fragments, 2.47
  numbered parts, 2.46, 8.121
  See also Greek; Latin
coauthors, 8.31–33, 8.89, 9.28–29, 10.4,
    10.6–8, 11.4–6
collected works, 11.13
colon, 3.88–90
  enumerations, 3.89, 3.109
  following, 3.89
  formal statement, 3.89
  glossary, 1.28
  hour and minute, 3.90
  legend, 7.16
  multivolume works, 8.80
  notes to tables, 6.51–52
  parenthetical references, 10.14
  periodical references, 8.99, 8.101
  place and publisher, 3.90, 8.55, 8.57
  with quotation marks, 3.106, 5.17
  scripture references, 2.21, 2.46, 3.90
  semicolon compared with, 3.88
  subtitle, 3.90, 4.6, 4.9–10, 8.39
  volume and page, 3.90, 8.70, 8.80,
    8.101, 10.14
color illustrations, 7.29, 7.30, 7.33
column headings (of tables), 6.33–38
  abbreviations, 6.35, 6.48–49
  capitalization, 6.38
  cut-in heads, 6.37, 6.38
  decked heads, 6.36–37, 14.28
  rules with, 6.36, 6.38
  runover lines, 6.38
  spacing, 6.38, 6.62
  spanner heads, 6.36, 6.38, 14.27
  for stub, 6.34, 6.39
  subheadings, 6.35, 6.38
  symbols, 6.48–49
comma, 3.65–83
  addresses, 2.66, 3.75
  adjectives preceding noun, 3.80
  adverbs, conjunctive, 3.76
  appositives, 3.73
  compound predicate, 3.67
  contrasting elements, 3.81
  dates, 2.49, 2.66
  degrees, 2.5
  interjections, 3.76
  levels of work, 2.46
  namely, that is, for example, i.e., e.g.,
    3.78
  notes, 8.24, 8.99

comma (*continued*)
  numbers, 2.66, 6.47
  with other punctuation, 3.104
  parenthetical elements, 3.77, 3.98
  phrases or clauses, 3.66, 3.72–73,
      3.78–79
  place-names, 3.75
  place of publication, 8.55
  to prevent misreading, 3.83
  with quotation marks, 3.106–7, 5.17
  restrictive and nonrestrictive clauses,
      3.72–73
  scholarly degrees, 2.5
  series, 3.68–71
  similar words, 3.82
  Sr., Jr., III, IV, 2.4
  title with name, 3.74
  versus semicolon, 3.84
  yet, so, 3.86
common nouns, possessives of, 3.9
company names, 2.12
compiler
  with author, 8.36, 8.40–42, 11.11
  author-date system, 10.3
  comp., 2.26
  in reference list, 10.31
components of works, 4.17, 8.25, 8.37–38,
      8.93, 10.28, 11.26–27
compositions (musical), 8.142–43,
      11.58–59
compound names, 9.17
compound predicate, 3.67
compounds, prepositional-phrase, 3.11
compounds, relationship, 3.13
compound sentences, 3.84–86
compound words, 3.12–34
  adjectives, 3.22–24, 3.27–33
  all, 3.26
  book, 3.20
  chemical terms, 3.25
  comparative forms, 3.23
  describing character, 3.18
  division, 3.47
  ed, 3.28
  elect, 3.17
  fold, 3.32
  fractions, 3.19
  house, 3.21
  like, 3.29
  nouns, 3.14–21
  numbers, 3.30–31
  odd, 3.30
  one word, 3.16
  personal names, 9.17
  prefixes, 3.34
  quasi, 3.33

relationships, 3.13
  See also division of words
computer graphics, 7.35, 13.21–23
  charts and graphs, 7.35, 13.21
  line drawings, 13.21
  maps, 7.34
  scanning images, 13.22
  vector graphics, 13.21–22
computer programs (software)
  block quotations, 5.5
  choosing, 13.3, 13.11
  citation of, 8.140, 11.57
  cross-references, 13.20
  cursor, 13.7
  ellipsis points, 3.59, 3.111, 5.18
  equations and formulas, 13.18
  footnotes, 13.17, 13.20, 14.17
  formatting functions, 13.15–16
  hyphenation and justification, 3.37,
      13.11, 13.16, 14.3
  indention, 14.4
  italics of underlining, 4.14
  note numbers, 5.5, 8.8, 8.13, 13.17
  printer interface, 13.25
  punctuation marks, 3.111
  rules, 13.19
  screen display, 13.7
  search and replace, 13.11
  special characters, 13.8
  stored keystrokes, 13.9
  style sheets, 13.12, 14.1
  superscripts, 13.17
  table of contents, 13.13
  tables, 6.2, 13.19
  text editing, 13.10–12
  word division, 3.37, 13.11, 13.16, 14.3
  See also computer graphics; computer
      systems
computer services, 8.141, 11.56–57, 12.20
computer systems
  backing up files, 13.14
  choosing, 13.2–6
  file management, 13.13
  printer, 13.24–30
  See also computer programs; printing
Congress, United States
  Congressional Information Service Index
      (*CIS/Index*), 12.7
  Congressional Record, 12.10, 12.12
  legislative publications, 12.8–12
conjunctions
  in compound sentences, 3.84–85
  coordinating, 3.66–69, 4.6–7
consonants, doubled, 3.41
constitutions, 2.27, 12.15, 12.21
content notes, 8.3, 8.149, 10.19, 14.38

continuation separator, 14.13
continued numers. *See* inclusive numbers
continued tables, 6.25
continuous-tone copy, 7.2–3, 7.35
coordinating conjunctions
    capitalization, 4.6–7
    compound predicates, 3.67
    with independent clauses, 3.66
    with series, 3.68–69
Copyright Act of 1976, 5.1
copyright date, 8.67–68
copyright notice, 1.8, 7.21
copyright page, 1.8, 1.11, 14.6
correcting and erasing, 13.31–34
correspondence. *See* letters (correspon-
        dence)
countries
    abbreviations, 2.13
    with public documents, 12.4
credit lines, 7.18–26
    content and style, 7.21
    courtesy, 7.24
    original material, 7.23–26
    placement, 7.20
    previously published material, 7.21–22
    public domain illustrations, 7.22
cross-hatching, 7.33
cross-references
    computer adjustment, 13.20
    multivolume works, 11.14
    in notes, 8.150–53
    with parenthetical references, 10.10,
        10.22, 11.2, 11.9, 12.1
    pseudonyms, 11.9
    public documents, 12.2, 12.8, 12.10,
        12.17, 12.19, 12.20, 12.21, 12.25
    reports, 11.33
currency
    British, 2.40–41, 3.51
    numbers for, 2.40–43
    U.S., 2.40–41, 3.52
cut-in heads (tables), 6.37–38

daisy wheel printers, 13.26, 13.28, 13.29
dash, 3.91–97
    in contents, 1.14
    before final clause, 3.95
    in glossary, 1.28
    interruptions, 3.93
    parenthetical material, 3.98
    repetition, 3.94
    sudden break in thought, 3.92
    typing, 3.91
    See also hyphen
date of publication, 8.67–69
    books, 8.67–69, 8.76–79

brackets with, 8.68, 11.54
from card catalog, 8.68
copyright date, 8.67
forthcoming, in press, 8.69
journals, 8.51, 8.101, 10.25
multivolume works, 8.76–79
n.d., 8.67, 10.25
in parenthetical references, 10.2, 10.11
public documents, 12.1
in reference lists, 10.25
uncertain, 11.54
dates
    centuries, 2.53
    copyright date, 8.67–68
    decades, 2.54
    eras, 2.56
    months, 2.49–51, 2.55, 3.51
    numbers in, 2.49–56
    word division, 3.51
    See also date of publication; day; year
day
    abbreviated, 2.55
    dates, 2.49–50
    time of day, 2.57
    word division, 3.51
decades, 2.54
decimals
    comma within, 2.66, 6.47
    currency, 2.40–42
    spelled out or numerals, 2.36
    in tables, 6.47
    zeros with, 2.36
decked heads, 6.36–37, 14.28
dedication, 1.9, 1.11, 14.6
degree (measure), 2.16–17, 6.43
degrees, scholarly, 2.5, 3.50
dependent clause, 3.72, 3.79
diacritical marks, 13.8
dictionaries, 3.1, 3.35, 8.51, 8.112
dimensions
    abbreviations, 2.16–17, 3.31
    pages, 13.35, 14.2
directions, in addresses, 2.15
display. *See* headings
dissertation bond paper, 13.30, 13.35,
        13.36
dissertations
    citation of, 4.19, 8.130, 11.55
    defined, 1.1
    microfilm reproduction of, 7.29, 8.2
distance, units of, 2.16–17
division of words, 3.35–53
    abbreviations, 3.50
    able and *ible,* 3.44
    capital letters, 3.50
    compounds, 3.47

division of words (*continued*)
  currency, 3.51
  dates, 3.51
  dictionaries, 3.1, 3.35, 3.48
  foreign languages, 3.53
  hyphenated words, 3.47
  ing or *ed,* 3.40–41
  initials, 3.49
  justification programs, 3.37, 13.11,
    13.16, 14.3
  one-letter divisions, 3.43
  by pronunciation, 3.38
  proper nouns, 3.48
  punctuation, 3.52
  suffixes, 3.45
  syllabication, 3.1, 3.35
  time, 3.51
  two-letter divisions, 3.46
  See also hyphenation
doctor (Dr.), 2.6
documentation, systems of, 11.1–68. *See
  also* bibliography; citation; notes;
  parenthetical references; reference
  list
documentation notes (reference notes),
  8.3, 8.21–22
documents. *See* electronic documents;
  public documents; unpublished
  material
dollar, 2.40
dollar sign ($), 2.40, 3.52, 6.43, 6.47
dot matrix printers, 13.28, 13.29
Dr. (doctor), 2.6
dry-mounting tissue, 7.38, 7.39, 7.42
duplicating, 13.36. *See also* photocopies
dynasties, 2.60

edited works, parts of, 4.17, 8.25, 8.37–38,
  8.93, 10.28, 11.26–27
editing text, 13.10–12
editions
  of classical works, 8.124
  documentation systems compared,
    11.18–20
  first, full reference, 8.44–48
  microform, 8.137–38, 11.51
  named, 8.47
  numbered, 8.45, 8.124
  paperback, 8.47, 11.20
  reprint, 8.46–47, 8.63, 11.19–20
editor, 8.40–42
  as author, 8.36, 11.11
  documentation systems compared,
    11.11, 11.12, 11.14, 11.17, 11.34
  ed., 2.26, 8.40–42, 10.31
  in parenthetical references, 10.3

series editor, 11.17
  See also compiler
editorial method (part of work), 1.13,
  1.31
Educational Resources Information Center (ERIC), 8.139, 12.5
e.g., 2.23, 2.26, 3.78
electronic documents, 8.141, 11.57, 12.1,
  12.20
ellipsis points
  computer formatting, 3.59, 3.111, 5.18
  with enumeration, 5.25
  faltering speech, 3.94
  in foreign language, 5.29
  full line of, 5.24–25
  omitting, 5.27–28
  with poetry, 5.24
  punctuation with, 5.20–23
  quotation marks with, 5.18
  with quotations, 5.18–28, 5.33–34
  spacing of, 5.18
em dash. *See* dash
emperors, 2.58
encyclopedias, citation of, 8.51, 8.112,
  11.42–43
end matter. *See* back matter
endnotes, 1.46, 8.2, 8.4, 8.15, 14.38. *See
  also* notes
enumerations
  ellipsis points, 5.25
  numbers, 2.70–71, 3.98
  parentheses, 2.70–71, 3.98
  punctuation, 3.57, 3.109
  quoting, 5.14
  See also lists
epigraph, 1.10–11, 5.9, 14.6
equations, 2.65, 13.2, 13.15, 13.18, 14.34
eras, 2.56
erasing, 13.31–34
ERIC (Educational Resources Information Center), 8.139, 12.5
essays, 4.17, 8.93. *See also* articles (periodical); chapters, citation of
et al., 2.26, 10.6–8
etc., 2.23, 2.26, 3.70
et seq., 2.26
evangelists, 2.9
exclamation point, 3.63–64
  with ellipsis points, 5.22
  with quotation marks, 3.106, 5.17

f., ff., 8.71
facts of publication
  for classical works, 8.51, 8.123
  in credit line, 7.21
  date of publication, 8.67–69

brackets with, 8.68, 11.54
from card catalog, 8.68
copyright date, 8.67
forthcoming, in press, 8.69
multivolume works, 8.76–79
n.d., 8.67, 10.25
in parenthetical references, 10.2,
10.11
periodicals, 8.101
public documents, 8.51, 12.1
in reference lists, 10.25
uncertain, 11.54
first, full reference, 8.51–69
items included, 8.24, 8.51, 8.66
n.p., 8.55–56
omissions, 8.51, 8.66, 11.42
place of publication, 8.52–56, 8.106–9
cities not widely known, 8.53
foreign cities, 8.54, 8.98, 8.108
newspapers, 8.106–9
punctuation with, 3.90, 8.55, 8.57
publisher, 8.57–66
copublished works, 8.60
foreign publishers, 8.65
omission in scientific fields, 8.66
reprint editions, 8.63
spelling and punctuation, 8.58–59
subsidiary, 8.61
reference books, 8.51, 11.42
in reference lists, 10.25, 10.32
fair use, 5.1
family names. *See* personal names
Federal Register, 12.13
figure numbers, 7.13–15
arabic numerals, 1.19, 7.13
and figure placement, 7.4
with legends, 7.8, 7.10
lettered parts in, 1.21, 7.8
in list of illustrations, 1.19–21
placement, 7.7, 7.12
figures. *See* illustrations; numbers; numerals
files (computer), 13.13–14
first, full reference (in notes), 8.21–22
bibliography entry compared with, 9.7
books, 8.22, 8.23–83
author, 8.26–36
author of preface, foreword, or introduction, 8.43, 11.24
edition, 8.44–48
editor, translator, or compiler, 8.36,
8.40–42, 11.11
facts of publication, 8.51–69
multivolume works, 8.74–83
page references, 8.70–73
series, 8.49–50

shortened title, 8.96 (*see also* shortened references)
title of work, 8.37–39, 8.80–81
newspaper articles, 8.105–10
periodical articles, 8.22, 8.97–110
fl., 2.26
folding illustrations, 7.5, 7.44–46
footnotes, 1.4
beginning of, 14.13
in block quotation, 14.16
endnotes compared with, 1.46, 8.2
indention, 14.13–14
layout on page, 8.15, 14.5, 14.13–17,
14.21
note numbers, 8.7–14, 14.13–14
within quotation, 14.16
sample pages with, 14.35, 14.36
separator, 8.15, 14.13
on short page, 14.15
software for entering, 5.5, 8.8, 8.13,
13.17, 13.19–20, 14.17
spacing, 1.2, 8.15, 14.5, 14.13–14,
14.17, 14.21
to tables, 6.50–58, 13.19, 14.29–30
See also notes
foreign languages
alphabetizing names, 9.18–22
anglicized words, 4.32
capitalization of titles, 4.10–12, 8.120,
9.35, 11.25
citing works in, 8.19–27, 9.35, 11.25
italics for, 2.25, 4.28–33, 9.35, 11.25
missing letters, 3.96
quotations in, 4.29–30, 5.29
translations, 4.33, 11.25
word division, 3.53
See also Greek; Latin
foreword, 4.13, 8.43, 11.24
for example, 2.23, 2.26, 3.78
formatting text
computer functions, 13.15–16
ellipsis points and leaders, 3.59, 3.111,
5.18
sample layouts, 14.1–42
See also layout
forms of address (social titles), 2.1, 2.3–
10, 4.31, 8.34
formulas, 2.65, 13.2, 13.15, 13.18, 14.34
forthcoming, 8.69
fractions
currency, 2.40–42
decimal, 2.36, 2.66, 6.47
hyphenation of, 3.19
spelled out or numeral, 2.36, 2.39
fragments, 2.47–48
fraternal lodges, 2.62, 2.66

French titles, capitalization of, 4.10
frontispiece, 14.7
front matter (preliminaries), 1.3, 1.7–32
    blank pages in, 1.8, 1.11, 14.6
    copyright page, 1.8, 1.11, 14.6
    dedication, 1.9, 1.11, 14.6
    pagination, 1.4–11, 8.70, 8.83, 14.6–7
    references to, 4.13, 8.70, 8.83
    in table of contents, 1.13, 14.19
    See also epigraph; glossary; list of ab-
        breviations; list of illustrations;
        list of tables; preface; table of
        contents; title page

geographical names
    abbreviations, 2.13–15
    capitalization, 4.1
    commas in, 3.75
    italics, 4.31
    See also political divisions
glossary, 1.13, 1.28–30, 14.33
government, 2.11, 2.60. *See also* political
    divisions; public documents
graphics. *See* computer graphics; illustra-
    tions
graphs
    computer graphics, 7.35, 13.21–23
    preparation, 7.30–31
    text reference, 7.4
Great Britain. *See* British currency; Brit-
    ish public documents
Greek
    capitalization of titles, 4.11, 8.120
    classical works, 2.22, 2.46–47, 8.51,
        8.119–27
    names of letters, 7.17
    possessives of names, 3.8

halftone copy, 7.2–3, 7.35. *See also* photo-
    graphs
Hansard's, 12.28
headings
    capitalization, 1.16, 4.6–7
    chapters, 1.13–15, 1.34, 1.36, 11.26–27,
        14.10, 14.34, 14.36
    in end matter, 1.39, 1.41, 1.46, 9.2,
        14.33, 14.39
    in front matter, 1.11, 1.19, 1.25–27,
        14.21, 14.22
    page numbers with, 14.8
    parts, 1.17, 1.35
    punctuation with, 1.37, 3.58, 8.39
    in quotations, 5.15
    spacing, 1.37, 14.5, 14.10
    in table of contents, 1.11–18
    See also column headings; subheads

headline-style capitalization, 1.23, 4.4–8,
    6.27–28, 6.38, 8.100, 10.27, 10.30,
    14.21
hellenized names, 3.8
hence, 3.86
Her (His) Majesty's Stationery Office
    (HMSO), 12.24
highway numbers, 2.63
homographs, 3.34
however, 3.86
hundred, 2.29
hyphen
    for dash, 2.91
    in inclusive numbers, 2.46, 2.67
    for missing letters or words, 3.96–97
    See also division of words; hyphenation
hyphenation
    adjectival compounds, 3.22–24, 3.27–33
    all, 3.26
    better, best, ill, lesser, little, well, 3.23
    centuries, 2.53
    chemical terms, 3.25
    compound words, 3.12–34
    fold, 3.32
    fractions, 3.19
    like, 3.29
    noun compounds, 3.14–21
    prefixes, 3.34
    quasi, 3.33
    relationship compounds, 3.13
    trend away from, 3.34
    See also division of words; hyphen

ibid., 2.23, 2.26, 8.85–87
id., 2.26, 8.86
idem, 8.86, 8.87
i.e., 2.23, 2.26, 3.78
illustrations (artwork), 7.1–46
    in appendix, 1.39, 7.4
    broadside, 7.9, 14.24
    captions (*see* captions)
    charts, 7.4, 7.30, 13.21
    color, 7.29, 7.30, 7.33
    from commercial agency, 7.25
    computer graphics, 7.34–35, 13.21–23
    continuous-tone copy, 7.2–3, 7.35
    credit lines, 7.18–26
    cross-hatching, 7.33
    duplicating, 13.36
    folding, 7.5, 7.44–46
    full-page, 7.5–6
    graphs, 7.4, 7.30–31, 7.35, 13.21–23
    grouped, 7.8, 7.9
    identifying parts, 7.16–17
    key, 7.11, 7.17
    line copy, 7.2–3, 7.29, 13.21

maps, 7.5, 7.10–11, 7.33–34, 7.44, 14.24
margins, 7.7
mounting, 7.37–43
numbering (*see* figure numbers)
page numbers with, 7.5–6, 7.7, 7.9
permissions, 7.18–22
photographs, 7.2, 7.29, 7.36–37
position, 7.4–12, 14.23
preparation, 7.27–46
public domain, 7.22
reduction, 7.32, 7.35
scale, 7.11
See also computer graphics; figure numbers; legends; list of illustrations
imperatives, 3.55
impressions (printings), 11.18
inclusive numbers (continued numbers)
hyphens between, 2.46, 2.67
page references, 2.67, 8.70–73
years, 2.67
indeed, 3.86
indention, 14.4
bibliography, 9.8
block quotations, 5.4, 5.30, 5.32, 14.4
enumerations, 2.72
footnotes, 14.13
outlines, 2.73
paragraph, 5.30, 14.4, 14.13
poetry, 5.7, 14.4
runover lines, 1.14, 1.24, 6.39
table of contents, 1.13–14
tables, 6.27–28, 6.38–39, 6.41, 6.46
independent clauses, 3.66, 3.72
indirect questions, 3.55
information services, 8.139, 11.56, 12.5, 12.7, 12.20
infra, 2.26, 8.151
initial numbers, 2.32–35
initials
authors' names, 2.2, 8.26, 14.39
word division, 3.49
in press, 8.69
interjections, 3.76
international bodies, documents of, 12.33
International System of Units (*Système international d'unités;* SI), 2.17
interpolations in quotations, 3.99, 5.35–37
interviews, 8.118, 11.48–50
introduction
citation of, 8.43, 11.24
editorial method in, 1.31
pagination, 1.34
position of, 1.34–35
references to, 4.13
inversion of author's name, 9.9–10
issue numbers, 8.101

italics
added for emphasis, 5.38
foreign words and phrases, 2.25, 4.28–33, 9.35
Latin terms, 2.23, 2.25, 2.26, 5.36, 8.85
legal cases, 4.22, 8.135
printing, 13.27
punctuation following, 4.14
ship, aircraft, and spacecraft, 4.26
titles of works, 4.14–27
books and periodicals, 4.16, 8.38, 9.34, 9.35, 11.25
foreign works, 9.35, 11.25
long poems, 4.16, 4.23, 8.115
motion pictures, 4.24
plays, 4.24
underlining for, 4.14, 5.38, 9.34, 11.21, 13.27

Japanese names, 9.21
Jesus, possessive of, 3.8
journals
abbreviation of titles, 8.19
citation of
book reviews, 8.117, 11.46
documentation systems compared, 11.39–40
first, full reference, 8.99–103
in reference lists, 10.25
subsequent references, 8.111
year of publication, 8.101
magazines compared with, 8.97
See also articles (periodical); periodicals
justification, computerized, 3.37, 13.11, 13.16, 14.3

key (to illustration), 7.11, 7.17
keys, musical, 4.7

labor unions, 2.62
laser printers, 13.28–29
Latin
capitalization of titles, 4.11–12, 8.120
classical works, 8.119–27
italics for, 2.23, 2.25, 2.26, 5.36, 8.85
law
abbreviations, 2.27, 8.87, 8.135
constitutions and bylaws, 2.27, 12.15, 12.21
idem, 8.87
infra and *supra,* 2.26, 8.151
legal cases, 4.22, 8.135
legal citations, 8.51, 8.133–35, 8.151
Uniform System of Citation, 8.133
See also legislative publications; public documents

layout
  footnotes, 8.15, 14.5, 14.13–17, 14.21
  illustrations (*see* illustrations)
  samples of, 14.1–42
  text, 13.15–16, 14.2–17
leaders. *See* period leaders
League of Nations, documents of, 12.33
lectures, 8.130
legal cases, 4.22, 8.135. *See also* law
legends, 7.10, 7.13–26
  capitalization and punctuation, 1.23,
    3.58, 7.14, 14.21
  and caption, 7.14
  credit lines in, 7.18–26
  figure numbers, 1.21, 7.8, 7.10
  grouping, 7.8–9
  identifying parts of illustration, 7.8,
    7.16–17
  and key, 7.17
  in list of illustrations, 1.22–23
  placement, 7.7–10, 7.12, 7.14, 7.15
  spacing, 7.15, 14.5
  See also illustrations
legislative publications
  British Parliamentary Papers, 12.26–28
  Canadian Parliament, 12.32
  United States Congress, 12.8–12
letters (of the alphabet)
  capitals, 2.11, 3.5, 3.6, 3.50
  with figure numbers, 1.21
  Greek, 7.17
  as keys to illustrations, 7.8, 7.16–17
  missing, 3.96–97
  plurals, 3.6
letters (correspondence)
  citation of, 8.4, 11.52
  quoting, 5.13
  as unpublished material, 8.130
libraries, 8.68, 8.131–32
like, 3.29
line copy, 7.2–3, 7.29, 13.21
lines
  line, 2.26, 8.114–15, 8.116
  numbers beginning, 2.72
  plays and poems, 8.114–16
  See also runover lines
list of abbreviations, 1.2, 1.13, 1.27, 14.32
list of illustrations, 1.2, 1.13, 1.19–23,
  14.21
list of references. *See* reference list
list of tables, 1.2, 1.13, 1.24, 14.22
lists, 1.2, 3.57, 3.89, 8.4. *See also* enumerations; list of abbreviations; list of illustrations; list of tables; reference
  list
loanwords, 4.32

local government documents (U.S.), 12.21
loc. cit., 8.84
lodges, fraternal, 2.62, 2.66
loose-leaf services, 8.139, 12.5

magazines
  documentation systems compared,
    11.41
  first, full reference, 8.104
  journals compared with, 8.97
  in reference lists, 10.25
  subsequent references, 8.111
  See also articles (periodical); period-
    icals
manuscript collections, 4.15, 4.20, 8.131–
  32, 10.16. *See also* unpublished
  manuscripts
maps, 7.5, 7.10–11, 7.33–34, 7.44, 14.24
margins
  for illustrations, 7.7
  ragged right, 3.37, 13.11, 13.16, 14.3
  for text, 14.2–3
mathematical text, 2.65, 13.2, 13.15,
  13.18, 14.34
measure, units of, 2.16–17, 2.64, 3.31
medieval works, 2.46, 8.51, 8.128
microfilming
  of computer graphics, 7.35
  of dissertations and theses, 7.29, 8.2
  of tables, 6.23
microform editions, 8.137–38, 11.51
midnight, 2.57
military divisions, 2.60
military titles, 2.7–8
million, 2.29, 2.35
missing letters or words, 3.96–97
monarchs, 2.58
money. *See* currency
month, 2.49–51, 2.55, 3.51
Moses, possessive of, 3.8
motion pictures, 4.24, 8.145, 11.61
mounting illustrations, 7.37–43
multiauthor works, 8.31–33, 8.89, 9.28–
  29, 10.4, 10.6–8, 11.4–6
  parts of, 4.17, 8.25, 8.37–38, 8.93,
    10.28, 11.26–27
multiple punctuation, 2.103–10. *See also*
  names of punctuation marks
multiple references, 8.16, 11.65–68
multivolume works
  cross-references to, 11.14
  date of publication, 8.76–79
  different titles, 8.81
  documentation systems compared,
    11.14–15
  first, full reference, 8.74–83

page references, 8.80–83
same title, 8.80
shortened references, 8.92
music
compositions, 4.7, 8.143
key symbols, 4.7
performances, 8.146, 11.47
recordings, 8.144
scores, 8.142, 11.58–59

namely, 3.78
names. *See* author's name; editor; geographical names; personal names;
proper nouns; publisher's name; titles of works
National Technical Information Service
(NTIS), 8.139, 12.5
n.d., 2.26, 8.67, 10.25
newspapers
American, 8.106–7
city of publication, 8.106–9
documentation systems compared,
11.44–45
first, full reference, 8.105–10
foreign, 8.108
microform, 8.138
in reference lists, 10.25
reviews, 8.117, 11.47
sections, 8.105
subsequent references, 8.111
the with title, 8.110
See also articles (periodical)
non-Latin alphabets, 7.17, 13.2, 13.8
nonrestrictive clauses, 3.72–73
noon, 2.57
note numbers, 8.7–14, 14.14
arabic numerals, 1.46, 8.7
computer programs, 5.5, 8.8, 8.13,
13.17
double, 8.14
endnotes, 1.46, 8.10, 8.15, 14.38
footnotes, 8.10, 14.13–14
position in text, 8.11
punctuation with, 1.46, 8.9, 14.14,
14.38
sequence, 8.12, 8.15, 13.17
superscript or on line, 8.8–10, 13.17,
14.14
notes, 8.1–153
abbreviations in, 2.12–13, 2.23, 2.26,
8.17–20
Apocrypha, 8.129
artworks, 8.147, 11.63–64
author-date system with, 10.19
author's name (*see* author's name)
Bible, 8.51, 8.129

bibliography entries compared with,
9.7–13, 11.1–68
books (*see* books, citation of)
capitalization of titles, 4.5–138, 8.120,
11.25
classical works, 8.119–27
computer programs, 8.140
computer services, 8.141, 12.20
content notes, 8.3, 8.149, 10.19, 14.38
cross-references, 8.3, 8.150–53
documentation (reference) notes, 8.3,
8.21–22
documentation systems compared, 9.7–
13, 11.1–68
electronic documents, 8.141, 11.57,
12.1, 12.20
encyclopedias and dictionaries, 8.51,
8.112, 11.42–43
endnotes (*see* endnotes)
first, full reference, 8.21–83, 8.97–110
footnotes (*see* footnotes)
interviews, 8.118, 11.48–50
legal citations, 8.51, 8.133–35, 8.151
lists in, 8.4
loose-leaf or information services,
8.139, 12.5, 12.7, 12.20
manuscript collections, 4.20, 8.131–32
medieval works, 8.51, 8.128
microform editions, 8.137–38, 11.51
multiple references, 8.16, 11.65–68
music, 8.142–44, 11.58–59
newspapers, 8.105–11, 8.138, 11.44–45
novels, 8.113
numbering (*see* note numbers)
page references (*see* page references)
pagination of, 14.8
performances, 8.146, 11.62
periodicals, 8.11, 8.99–104, 11.39–41
plays, 8.114–15
poems, 8.114–16
position, 8.15–16
public documents, 8.83, 8.134, 8.136,
12.1–33
punctuation in, 3.90, 8.55, 8.57, 8.70,
9.11, 10.14
quotations containing, 8.5
quotations in, 5.10
recordings, 8.144–45, 11.60–61
reducing, 8.16
reviews, 8.117, 11.46–47
scriptures, 8.51, 8.129
secondary sources, 8.148
shortened references (*see* shortened references)
spacing, 1.2, 8.15, 14.5, 14.13–14,
14.17, 14.21

notes (*continued*)
  subsequent references (*see* subsequent
    references)
  tables in, 8.4
  to tables, 6.28, 14.29, 14.30
  translations in, 4.33, 11.25
  unpublished material, 8.83, 8.130–32,
    11.52–57
  See also citation; endnotes; first, full ref-
    erence; footnotes; note numbers;
    page references; parenthetical
    references; subsequent refer-
    ences
nouns, 3.7–10, 3.14–15, 3.80. *See also*
  proper nouns
novels, 8.113
n.p., 2.26, 8.55, 8.56
NTIS (National Technical Information
  Service), 8.139, 12.5
numbers, 2.29–73
  alignment, 2.72, 6.46–47
  beginning sentence, 2.32, 2.72
  cardinal, 2.30, 3.30, 3.31
  church names, 2.61
  commas within, 2.66, 6.47
  in compound words, 3.30, 3.31
  currency, 2.40–43, 3.51
  dates, 2.49–56
  decimals, 2.36, 2.40–42, 2.66, 6.43–44,
    6.47
  enumerations, 2.70–72, 3.57, 3.98
  fractions, 2.36, 2.39, 2.40–42, 3.19, 6.47
  general rule, 2.29–30
  government designations, 2.60
  highway numbers, 2.63
  hundred, 2.29
  lodges and unions, 2.62, 2.66
  monarchs, 2.58
  ordinal, 2.30
  with parenthetical references, 2.71,
    10.33–34
  part numbers, 1.13, 1.17, 1.35
  parts of works, 2.44–48
  percentages, 2.36–38, 6.5, 6.47
  with personal names, 2.58–59
  plurals, 2.68–69
  round numbers, 2.29, 2.34–35, 2.41
  in scientific writing, 2.64–65
  series (works), 8.50
  series of numbers, 2.31–33
  spelled out or numerals, 2.29–64
  street addresses, 2.63
  superscript, 8.8–10, 13.17, 14.14
  telephone numbers, 2.63, 2.66
  thousand, 2.29
  time of day, 2.57

volume and issue numbers, 8.78–83,
  8.92, 8.101, 8.104, 11.14–15
whole numbers, 2.36, 2.40
zero, 2.36, 2.40, 6.43–44
See also chapter numbers; figure numbers; fractions; inclusive numbers; mathematical text; note
  numbers; numerals; page numbers; table numbers
numerals
  alignment, 2.72, 6.46–47
  commas within, 2.66, 6.47
  currency, 2.40–43, 3.51
  dates, 2.50, 2.54, 2.56
  decimals and percentages, 2.36, 2.40–
    42, 2.66, 6.43–44, 6.47
  fractions, 2.36, 2.39, 2.40–42, 3.19
  general rule for numbers, 2.29–30
  spelled out or numerals, 2.29–64
  percentages, 2.36–38, 6.5, 6.47
  plurals, 2.68
  round numbers, 2.34–35
  series of numbers, 2.31–33
  time of day, 2.57
  See also arabic numerals; numbers; roman numerals

on-line materials. *See* electronic documents
op. cit., 8.84
ordinal numbers, 2.30
organization names, 2.11–12
outlines, 2.73, 5.14, 5.24, 8.4

p., pp., 2.26, 8.70, 10.13
page numbers (pagination), 1.4, 14.6–9
  acknowledgments, 1.26
  arabic numerals, 1.4, 14.8
  back matter, 1.3–4, 1.44, 14.8
  bibliographies, 14.8
  blank page or copyright page, 1.8, 14.6
  broadside pages, 6.22, 7.9, 14.24, 14.30
  dedication, 1.9, 1.11, 14.6
  epigraph, 1.10, 14.6
  frontispiece, 14.7
  front matter, 1.4–11, 8.70, 8.83, 14.6–7
  with illustrations, 7.5–6, 7.7, 7.9, 14.24
  introduction, 1.34
  with legends, 7.8
  in list of illustrations, 1.19–20, 14.21
  in list of tables, 1.24, 14.22
  with major heading, 14.8
  notes section, 14.8
  photocopies in appendixes, 1.44
  position, 7.8, 14.7–9
  roman numerals, 1.4, 1.26, 14.7

in table of contents, 1.14, 1.18
tables, 6.22, 14.30
text, 1.4, 14.8
title page, 1.7, 14.6, 14.7
See also page references
page references (citation)
arabic numerals, 8.83
articles in periodicals, 8.71–72
in bibliographies, 9.12–13
books, 8.70–73
f., ff., 8.71
first, full reference, 8.70–73
inclusive numbers, 2.67, 8.70–73
multivolume works, 8.80–83
p., pp., 2.26, 8.70, 10.13
parenthetical references, 10.12–14
passim, 2.26, 8.73
preliminaries, 8.83
public documents, 8.83
punctuation, 2.66, 3.90, 8.70, 8.101,
10.14
roman numerals, 8.83
See also page numbers
pages
dimensions, 13.35, 14.2
format, 1.38, 13.15–16, 14.1–42
See also broadside pages; layout; margins; page numbers
pamphlets, 4.16, 8.49–50
paper, 13.4, 13.35
acid-free stock, 13.28, 13.33, 13.35,
13.36
dissertation bond, 13.30, 13.35, 13.36
photocopying, 13.35, 13.36
paperback editions, 8.47, 11.20
paragraphs
in block quotations, 5.4, 5.30, 5.33,
14.37
indention, 5.30, 14.4, 14.13
numbers beginning, 2.72
omission of, 5.33
para., 2.26
parentheses, 3.98
with abbreviations, 1.27
bibliographies, 9.11
versus brackets, 3.99, 5.35
with enumerations, 2.70–71, 3.98
and line breaks, 3.52
multiple punctuation, 3.105, 3.108–9
notes, 8.24, 9.11
with parenthetical elements, 3.98
with parenthetical references, 10.2,
10.18
with source, 3.98, 7.20
table of contents, 1.18
with translation, 4.33, 11.25

parenthetical elements, 3.77, 3.98–99,
3.108
parenthetical references, 8.1, 8.4, 10.1–19
abbreviations, 2.12, 2.18, 2.23
artworks, 11.63–64
author-date system, 10.2–19, 12.2,
12.21
author's name, 10.2–11, 10.18, 11.13–15
with block quotation, 5.30
books, 11.3–38
cross-references, 8.4, 8.150, 10.10,
10.22, 11.2, 12.1
date of publication, 10.2, 10.11
in dissertations, 1.46
documentation systems compared,
11.1–68
encyclopedias, 11.42–43
interviews, 11.48–50
microform editions, 11.51
MLA system, 8.1
multiple references, 10.11–12, 11.67
music, 11.58–59
newspapers, 11.44–45
with numbers, 2.17, 10.33–34
page references, 10.12–14
performances, 11.62
periodicals, 11.39–41
placement of, 10.18
public documents, 12.1–33
publisher, 10.9–10
punctuation in, 10.3, 10.7, 10.12, 10.14
recordings, 11.60–61
reviews, 11.46–47
unpublished materials, 11.52–57
volume number, 10.14
See also citation; reference list
Parliamentary Debates (U.K.), 12.28
Parliamentary Papers (U.K.), 12.26–27
particles, names with, 9.15
parts (sections of paper), 1.35
numbers, 1.13, 1.17, 1.35
part-title page, 1.35, 14.6
in table of contents, 1.13, 1.17–18
titles, 1.13, 1.15, 14.19, 14.20
parts of a work
abbreviations, 2.18, 8.18
citation of, 2.44–48, 4.17, 8.25, 8.37–
38, 8.43, 8.70, 8.83, 8.93, 10.28,
11.24, 11.26–27
text references to, 2.18, 4.1, 4.13, 8.18,
8.37
See also chapters
passim, 2.26, 8.73
percentage, 2.36–38, 3.31, 6.5, 6.31
performances, 8.146, 11.47, 11.62
period, 3.55–59

period (*continued*)
  with abbreviations, 2.2, 2.3, 2.11, 3.6,
    3.56, 3.103, 8.19
  bibliographies, 8.99, 9.11
  classical references, 2.46, 8.121
  and computer programs, 3.59, 3.111,
    5.18
  with ellipses, 3.59, 5.18, 5.27
  in glossary, 1.28
  legends, 3.58, 7.14
  with note numbers, 1.46, 8.9, 14.14,
    14.38
  notes, 8.19, 8.24, 8.99
  with numbers, 2.72, 3.57
  when omitted, 2.2, 3.57–58, 8.9, 8.19
  with parentheses or brackets, 3.108
  questions, 3.55, 3.61
  with quotation marks, 3.106, 3.107,
    5.17
  reference lists, 10.23
  scripture references, 2.21, 2.46, 8.129
  social titles, 2.3
  statements, 3.55
  subheadings, 3.58
  in table of contents, 1.14
  table titles, 3.58, 6.27
  See also ellipsis points; period leaders
periodicals, 8.97–111
  city, 8.98, 8.106–9
  date, 8.22, 8.51, 8.97, 8.101, 10.25
  facts of publication, 8.51, 8.97–98
  foreign, 8.98, 8.108, 8.100, 8.110
  series, 8.102
  titles, 4.16, 8.19, 8.98, 8.106, 8.108,
    8.100, 8.110, 9.34, 10.30
  types of, 8.97
  volume and issue numbers, 8.22, 8.97,
    8.101, 8.104
  See also articles (periodical); journals;
    magazines; newspapers
period leaders
  computer formatting, 3.59
  list of illustrations, 1.19
  table of contents, 1.18
  tables, 3.59, 6.42, 6.45
permissions
  in acknowledgments, 1.26
  credit lines, 7.18–26
  fair use, 5.1
  illustrations, 7.18–22
  public domain, 7.22
  quotations, 5.1
  table data, 6.51
personal names
  alphabetizing, 9.14–26, 9.32
  Arabic, 9.19

capitalization, 4.1–2
Chinese, 9.20
compound, 9.17
family names, 9.23–24
foreign, 4.31, 9.18–22
initials in, 2.2, 3.49, 8.26, 14.39
Japanese, 9.21
Mc, M, Mac, 9.15–16
  with particles, 9.15
  plurals, 3.2–4
  possessives, 3.7, 3.8, 3.10
  pseudonyms, 8.27–29, 9.26, 11.9
  religious names and titles, 1.7–8, 9.25
  Saint, 2.9–10, 9.16
  Spanish, 9.18
  Sr., Jr., III, IV, 2.4, 2.59, 9.24
  titles with, 2.1, 2.3–10, 4.31, 8.34
  word division, 3.48
  See also author's name
phonetic transcriptions, 3.100
photocopies
  correcting, 13.33–34
  documents in appendixes, 1.44
  paper for, 13.35, 13.36
  quality, 13.4
photographs, 7.2, 7.29, 7.36–37
phrases, introductory, 3.79
place-names. *See* geographical names
place of publication, 8.52–56, 8.106–9
  cities not widely known, 8.53
  foreign cities, 8.54, 8.98, 8.108
  newspapers, 8.106–9
  punctuation, 3.90, 8.55, 8.57
plagiarism, 5.2
plays
  note references, 8.114–15
  reviews, 8.117, 11.47
  titles, 4.24
plurals
  abbreviations, 2.26, 3.6
  letters, 3.5, 3.6
  numbers, 2.68–69
  personal names, 3.2–4, 3.10
  possessives, 3.10
  prepositional-phrase compounds, 3.11
P.M., 2.57
poetry
  ellipses with, 5.24
  indention of, 5.7, 14.4
  line breaks, 5.8
  note references, 8.114–16
  quotations, 5.6–8, 5.10, 14.37
  shortened references, 8.93
  spacing, 5.6
  titles, 4.16, 4.23, 8.115–16, 11.22, 11.28
political divisions

cities and towns, 8.53, 8.54, 12.4
countries, 2.13, 12.4
  numbers in names of, 2.60
  public documents, 12.4
  states, 2.13, 12.4
popes, 2.58
possessives, 3.7–11
predicate, compound, 3.67
preface, 1.25
  acknowledgments in, 1.25
  author of, 8.43, 11.24
  references to, 4.13
  source of illustrations in, 7.20
  in table of contents, 1.13
prefixes, 2.14, 3.34
preliminaries. *See* front matter; *and names
  of elements*
prepositional phrases, 3.11, 3.79
prepositions, capitalization of, 4.6–7
presidential documents, 12.13–14
press-apply tones, 7.29–30, 7.33
printing, 13.24–30
printings (impressions) of books, 11.18
privately printed books, 11.29–30
proceedings, 11.34–36
professional titles, 2.3–10
proper adjectives, 4.2–3
proper nouns
  capitalization, 4.1–3
  company names, 2.12
  italics, 4.31
  plurals, 3.2–4
  possessives, 3.7–10
  word division, 3.48
  See also geographical names; personal
    names
prose, quotation of, 5.4–5, 5.10, 14.37
pseudonyms, 8.27–29, 9.26, 11.9
publication, date of. *See* date of publication
publication, defined, 8.130
publication, facts of. *See* facts of publication
publication, place of. *See* place of publication
public documents
  agency name, 12.4
  author of, 12.4
  British, 12.22–31
  Canadian, 12.32
  card catalog information, 12.3
  citing, 8.83, 8.134, 8.136, 12.1–33
  cross-references, 12.2, 12.8, 12.10,
    12.17, 12.19, 12.20, 12.21, 12.25
  facts of publication, 8.51, 12.1
  international bodies, 12.33

issuing agency, 12.2
League of Nations, 12.33
numbered parts, 2.45
on-line materials, 12.1
page references, 8.83
place-name, 12.4
state and local government documents
  (U.S.), 12.21
United Kingdom, 12.22–31
United Nations, 12.33
United States (*see* United States government documents)
  See also constitutions
public domain, 7.22
*Public General Acts and General Synod
  Measures,* 12.25
publisher's name, 8.57–66
  copublished works, 8.60
  foreign publishers, 8.65
  omission of, 8.66
  reprint editions, 8.63
  spelling and punctuation of, 8.57–59
  subsidiary, 8.61
punctuation, 3.54–111
  bibliographies, 3.90, 8.55, 8.57, 9.11
  brackets, 3.105, 3.108, 3.110
  and computer programs, 3.111
  ellipsis points, 5.20–23
  enumerations, 3.109
  headings, 1.37, 3.58, 8.39
  hence, however, indeed, thus, yet, so, 3.86
  with italics, 4.14
  legends, 3.58, 7.14
  line breaks, 3.52
  multiple, 3.103–10
  namely, that is, for example, 3.78
  note numbers, 1.46, 8.9, 14.14, 14.38
  page numbers, 2.66, 3.90, 8.70, 8.101,
    10.14
  parentheses and brackets, 3.105,
    3.108–9
  parenthetical references, 10.3, 10.7,
    10.12, 10.14, 10.18
  place of publication, 3.90, 8.55, 8.57
  publisher's name, 3.90, 8.55, 8.57–58
  quotation marks, 3.105–7, 5.17
  titles and subtitles, 3.90, 8.37, 8.39
  See also names of punctuation marks

quasi, 3.33
question mark, 3.60–62
  with ellipsis points, 5.22
  queries, 3.60
  quotation marks with, 3.106, 5.17
  for uncertainty, 3.62, 11.54
questionnaires, 1.44

questions, 3.55, 3.60–61
quotation marks, 5.11–17
  ellipsis points with, 5.18
  fragments of quotation, 5.31
  in linguistics, philosophy, and theology,
    3.107, 5.12
  poetry, 5.8
  prose quotations, 5.4, 5.10
  punctuation with, 3.105–7, 5.17
  single, 3.107, 5.11–12, 5.16, 11.23
  titles of works, 4.14–27, 5.12, 8.38, 9.35
    articles, chapters, short stories, 4.17,
      8.38, 11.22, 11.28
    in bibliographies, 9.34
    dissertations, 4.19
    poems, 4.16, 4.23, 8.116, 11.22, 11.28
    title within title, 11.21–23
    unpublished works, 4.19, 11.36
quotations, 5.1–38
  accuracy, 5.3
  in appendix, 5.14
  block (*see* block quotations)
  brackets with, 3.99, 3.110, 5.35
  capitalization, 5.26, 5.30
  ellipsis points, 5.18–28, 5.33–34
  enumerations, 5.14
  fair use, 5.1
  footnotes in, 14.16
  in foreign languages, 4.29–30, 5.29
  headings and subheadings, 5.15
  interpolations, 3.99, 3.110, 5.35–37
  italics added, 5.38
  letters, 5.13
  in notes, 5.10
  omissions, 5.18–29, 5.33–34
  outlines, 5.14
  permissions, 5.1
  poetry, 5.6–8, 5.10, 14.37
  prose, 5.4–5, 5.10
  within quotations, 5.11, 5.16, 5.17
  reducing notes, 8.16
  secondary source, 11.31
  sic, 3.64, 5.36
  source, 3.98, 5.7, 5.9
  spacing, 1.2, 5.4, 5.6, 14.5
  spelling, 3.1
  See also block quotations; epigraph
q.v., 2.26

radio programs, 4.25
ragged right margin, 3.37, 13.11, 13.16
recordings, 8.144–45, 11.60–61
reference books, 8.51, 8.112, 11.42–43
reference list, 10.20–32
  abbreviations, 2.12–13, 10.30–31

alphabetizing, 10.20–21 (*see also under*
    bibliography)
arrangement of elements, 10.20–32
authors' names, 10.21–22, 10.24, 11.2,
    11.3–15 (*see also under* bibliog-
    raphy)
books, 10.26, 11.3–38
chapter titles, 10.28
constitutions, 12.21
cross-references, 10.22, 11.2, 11.9,
    11.14, 11.33, 12.2, 12.8, 12.10,
    12.17, 12.19, 12.20, 12.21, 12.25
date of publication, 10.23, 10.25
documentation systems compared,
    11.1–68
encyclopedias, 11.42–43
facts of publication, 10.25, 10.32 (*see
    also under* bibliography)
heading, 10.2
initials, 14.39
interviews, 11.48–50
microform editions, 11.51
multiple references, 11.68
multivolume works, 11.14
music, 11.58–59
newspapers, 11.44–45
numbered list, 2.71, 10.33–34
pagination, 14.8
performances, 11.62
periodicals, 10.25, 10.29–30, 11.39–41
pseudonyms, 11.9
public documents, 12.1–33
punctuation, 3.90, 10.23
recordings, 11.60–61
reprint editions, 11.19
reviews, 11.46–47
sample pages, 14.39, 14.40
titles of works, 10.26–30 (*see also under*
    bibliography)
unpublished materials, 11.52–57
works of art, 11.63–64
See also bibliography; parenthetical ref-
    erences
reference matter. *See* back matter
reference notes (documentation notes),
    8.3, 8.21–22
relationship compounds, 3.13
religious names and titles, 2.7–8, 9.25
reports and proceedings, 11.32–33, 11.36
reprint editions, 8.46–47, 8.63, 11.19–20
resolution, printer, 13.28
restrictive clauses, 3.72–73
reviews, 8.117, 11.46–47
romance languages, 4.10
roman numerals

chapter numbers, 1.17
monarchs, popes, and the like, 2.58
outlines, 2.73
page numbers, 1.4, 1.26, 8.83, 14.7
page references, 2.44, 8.83
part numbers, 1.17
round numbers, 2.29, 2.34–35, 2.41
rules (typographic)
  computer-generated, 13.19
  hand-drawn, 6.65
  separator for footnotes, 8.15, 14.13
  tables, 6.36, 6.38, 6.59–65, 13.19, 14.25,
    14.26
  typewriter, 6.64
  vertical, 6.65, 14.26
run-in subheads, 1.14, 1.18, 1.37, 14.11
runover lines
  glossary, 1.28
  indention, 1.14, 6.38, 6.39
  list of abbreviations, 1.27
  list of tables, 1.2, 1.24
  with numbers, 2.72
  poetry, 5.7
  spacing, 1.2, 1.13
  subheads, 1.2
  table of contents, 1.2, 1.13–14, 14.20
  tables, 6.38, 6.39, 6.46

Saint
  alphabetizing *St.,* 9.16
  geographical names, 2.14
  personal names, 2.9–10, 9.16
scale, with illustrations, 7.11
scanning images, 13.22
scholarly degrees, 2.5, 3.50
scholarship, abbreviations, 2.18–23
scientific and technical writing
  abbreviations, 2.17, 2.64–65, 8.17
  capitalization, 4.5
  chemical terms, 3.25, 6.28
  equations and formulas, 2.65, 13.18
  glossary, 1.28
  numerals, 2.64–65
  parenthetical references using numbers,
    10.33–34
  publisher, 8.66
  symbols, 2.64–65
  titles of works, 9.34
scores, musical, 8.142, 11.58–59
screen display, 13.7
scriptures, 2.20–21, 2.46–47, 3.90, 4.21,
    8.51, 8.129
search and replace operation, 13.11
second, 2.30
secondary sources, 8.148, 11.31

section, 2.27
sections, 1.15, 1.37–38
semicolon, 3.84–88, 3.106, 5.17, 11.6
sentence-style capitalization, 2.73, 4.5,
    4.9, 6.27, 6.38, 9.35, 10.26, 10.28–
    29, 11.25
separator (footnotes), 8.15, 14.13
serial comma, 3.68
series
  citation of, 4.15, 4.18, 8.49–50,
    11.16–17
  editor, 11.17
  numbered, 8.50
  old and new, 8.102
  periodical, 8.102
  radio and television, 4.25
series of numbers, 2.31, 2.33
Sessional Papers (U.K.), 12.27
ships, 4.26
shortened references (in notes), 8.88–98
  short titles, 8.20, 8.91–92, 8.94–96
  two methods, 8.88, 8.90, 8.91
short stories, 4.17, 11.22, 11.28
SI (*Système international d'unités;* Interna-
    tional System of Units), 2.17
sic, 2.25, 2.26, 3.64, 5.36
sidehead, 1.37, 14.11
slash, in poetry, 5.8
so, 3.86
social titles, 2.1, 2.3–10, 4.31, 8.34
software. *See* computer programs
sound recordings, 8.144, 11.60
sources
  illustrations, 7.18–26
  poetry, 5.7, 5.9
  quotations, 3.98, 5.7, 5.9
  secondary, 8.148, 11.31
  tables, 6.50–51, 14.29, 14.30
  See also credit lines
sovereigns, 2.58
spacecraft, 4.26
spacing
  appendix, 1.43
  bibliography, 1.2, 9.8
  block quotations, 1.2, 5.4, 5.6, 14.5
  computer needs, 13.17, 14.5
  footnotes, 1.2, 6.58, 14.5, 14.13–14,
    14.17, 14.21
  glossary, 1.28
  headings, 1.37, 14.5, 14.10
  legends, 7.15, 14.5
  list of abbreviations, 1.27
  list of illustrations, 1.2, 1.19
  list of tables, 1.2, 1.24
  lists, 1.2

spacing (*continued*)
  notes, 1.2, 6.58, 14.5, 14.13–14, 14.17, 14.21
  poetry, 5.6
  quotations, 1.2, 5.4, 5.6, 14.5
  runover lines, 1.2, 1.13
  tables of contents, 1.2, 1.13
  tables, 1.2, 6.19, 6.27–28, 6.38–39, 6.58, 6.62
  text, 14.5
Spanish names, 9.18
spanner heads, 6.36, 6.38, 6.60, 14.27
special characters, 7.17, 13.2, 13.8, 13.26
speeches, 8.130, 8.132, 11.53
spelling, 3.1–53, 8.58. *See also* compound words; division of words; numbers, spelled out or numerals; plurals; possessives
Sr., Jr., III, IV, 2.4, 2.59, 9.24
state and local documents, 12.21
state names, 2.13, 12.4
statistical tables. *See* tables
Statutes at Large, United States, 12.10–11
Statutes of Canada, 12.32
stored keystrokes, 13.9
street addresses
  abbreviations, 2.15
  comma in, 2.66, 3.75
  numerals, 2.63
  in quotations, 5.13
  zip codes, 2.66, 3.75
stub, 6.34, 6.39–42. *See also* tables
styles and style sheets, 13.12, 14.1
subheads
  bibliography, 9.3–5
  capitalization, 1.16
  centered, 1.37, 14.11
  levels, 1.37–38
  page layout, 1.38, 14.11–12, 14.31, 14.35
  punctuation, 1.37, 3.58
  in quotations, 5.15
  run-in, 1.14, 1.18, 1.37, 14.11
  runover lines, 1.2, 1.14
  sideheads, 1.37, 14.11
  spacing, 1.2
  in table of contents, 1.11, 1.12, 1.14, 1.18, 14.19, 14.20
  tables, 6.32, 6.35, 6.38
subsequent references (in notes), 8.20, 8.84–96, 8.111. *See also* shortened references
subtitles
  capitalization, 4.6, 10.26, 11.25
  foreign, 11.25
  punctuation, 3.90, 8.37, 8.39

shortened references, 8.92
suffixes, 3.29, 3.44–45
superscript numbers, 8.8–10, 13.17, 14.14
supra, 2.26, 8.151
s.v., 2.23, 2.26, 8.112, 11.42
syllabication, 3.1, 3.35. *See also* division of words
symbols
  in illustration keys, 7.17
  musical keys, 4.7
  scientific and mathematical texts, 2.64–65
  special characters, 7.17, 13.2, 13.8, 13.26
  tables, 6.43, 6.47, 6.48–49, 6.55–57
Système international d'unités (SI; International System of Units), 2.17

table numbers, 6.13–17
  arabic numerals, 1.24, 6.13, 6.28
  computer-generated, 13.19
  in list of tables, 1.24
  position, 6.27
table of contents, 1.11–18
  capitalization in, 1.15–16
  computer-generated, 13.13
  omissions, 1.9–11
  page numbers in, 1.14, 1.18
  part and chapter numbers in, 1.13, 1.17
  part titles in, 1.13, 1.15, 14.19, 14.20
  period leaders, 1.18
  runover lines, 1.2, 1.13–14, 14.20
  spacing, 1.2, 1.13
  subheads in, 1.11, 1.12, 1.14, 1.18, 14.19, 14.20
tables, 6.1–65
  alignment, 6.46–47
  in appendixes, 1.39, 6.14, 8.4
  arrangement of elements, 6.12–47
  blank cells, 6.45, 14.27
  broadside, 6.22, 14.30
  column headings (*see* column headings)
  computer software for, 6.2, 13.19
  continued, 6.25
  database, 6.5
  decimals in, 6.47
  dichotomies, 6.6, 6.7, 6.10, 6.11
  on facing pages, 6.23
  footnotes, 6.50–58, 13.19, 14.29, 14.30
  list of (*see* list of tables)
  long and narrow, 6.21
  note references to, 8.4
  with notes, 6.50–58, 13.19, 14.29, 14.30
  numbering (*see* table numbers)
  percentages in, 6.5, 6.31
  period leaders, 6.42

permissions for, 6.51
position, 6.18–20, 14.31
ruling, 6.35, 6.38, 6.59–65, 13.19, 14.25, 14.26
size and shape, 6.20–24
spacing, 1.2, 6.19, 6.27–28, 6.38–39, 6.58, 6.62
stub, 6.34, 6.39–42
text references, 6.13, 6.15–18
titles (*see* table titles)
totals, 6.41
variables, 6.4, 6.6
wide, 6.22–24
zeros in, 6.43–44
See also column headings; list of tables; stub; table numbers; table of contents; table titles
table titles, 6.13, 6.26–32
capitalization, 6.27–28
content, 6.29
grammatical form, 6.30–31
in list of tables, 1.24
position, 6.27
punctuation, 3.58, 6.27
subheadings, 6.32
technical reports, 12.20
technical terms, glossary for, 1.28
technical writing. *See* scientific and technical writing
telephone numbers, 2.63, 2.66
television programs, 4.25
text, 1.33–38
editing, 13.10–12
entering, 13.7–19
laying out, 13.15–16, 14.2–17
margins, 3.37, 13.11, 13.16, 14.2–3
pagination, 1.4, 14.8
spacing, 14.5
that is, 2.23, 2.26, 3.78
the, 4.6–7, 8.95, 8.110, 9.27, 9.31
then, 3.86
theses
citation of, 4.19, 11.55
defined, 1.1
microfilm reproduction of, 7.29, 8.2
third, 2.30
thousand, 2.29
thus, 3.86
TIAS (Treaties and Other International Acts), 12.18
time, 2.49–57
A.M. and P.M., 2.57
century, 2.53
of day, 2.57
day, month, and year, 2.49–52, 2.55
decade, 2.54

era, 2.56
hour and minute, 3.90
midnight and noon, 2.57
word division, 3.51
title page, 1.7, 1.11, 14.6–7, 14.18
titles (with names), 2.1, 2.3–10, 4.31, 8.34
titles of works
abbreviation of, 8.19–20
article with, 8.95, 8.110, 9.27, 9.31
with author's name, 8.42
in bibliographies, 4.5–13, 9.31, 9.34–35
bulletins, 4.16
capitalization, 4.5–13, 8.100, 8.120, 9.35, 10.26, 10.30, 11.25
first, full reference, 8.37–39, 8.80–81
foreign, 4.10–12, 8.120, 9.35, 11.25
Greek and Latin, 4.11–12, 8.120
ibid., 8.85
italics, 4.14–27, 8.38, 8.115, 9.34–35
motion pictures, 4.24
multivolume works, 8.80–81
pamphlets, 4.16, 8.49–50
parts of work, 4.17, 8.37, 9.34, 11.22, 11.27
plays, 4.24
poems, 4.16, 4.23, 8.115–16, 11.22, 11.28
punctuation, 3.90, 8.37, 8.39
quotation marks with, 4.14–27, 5.12, 8.38, 9.34–35, 11.21–23, 11.28
radio and television programs, 4.25
recordings, 8.144–45, 11.60–61
in reference lists, 10.26–30
scripture, 2.20–21, 4.21, 8.129
shortened references, 8.20, 8.91–92, 8.94–96
subtitles, 3.90, 4.6, 8.37, 8.39, 10.26, 11.25
title within title, 11.21–23
translation of, 11.25
unpublished material, 4.19, 8.131, 11.36
See also chapter titles
total, mean, average, 6.41
trade unions, 2.62
transitional adverbs, 3.86
translation
book title, 11.25
words in text, 4.33
translator
first, full reference, 8.40–42, 11.12
parenthetical references, 10.3, 10.31, 11.12
trans., 2.26, 10.31
treaties, 12.18
Treaties and Other International Acts (TIAS), 12.18

typefaces, 13.27
type size, 13.27
typewriter
    correcting typewritten papers, 13.32
    hyphens for dashes, 3.91
    rules, 6.64
    underlining, 4.14

underlining, 4.14, 5.38, 9.34, 11.21, 13.27.
    See also italics
Uniform System of Citation, 8.133
Union of Soviet Socialist Republics
    (USSR), 2.13
unions, labor, 2.62
United Kingdom. *See* British currency;
    British public documents
United Nations (UN), 12.33
United States currency, 2.40–41, 3.52,
    6.43, 6.47
United States government documents,
    12.5–20
    bills and resolutions, 12.10–11
    *Congressional Information Service In-
        dex,* 12.7
    Congressional Record, 12.10, 12.12
    Constitution, 12.15
    debates, 12.12
    executive department documents, 12.17
    Federal Register, 12.13
    government commissions, 12.16
    hearings, 12.9
    *Introduction to United States Public
        Documents,* 12.20
    legislative publications, 12.8–12
    *Monthly Catalog of United States Gov-
        ernment Publications,* 12.5
    presidential documents, 12.13–14
    published documents, 12.8–18
    technical reports, 12.20
    treaties, 12.18
    Traties and Other International Acts,
        12.18
    United States Code, 12.11
    United States Statutes at Large, 12.10,
        12.11
    *United Sttaes Treaties and Other Inter-
        national Agreements,* 12.18
    unpublished documents, 12.19
    *Weekly Compilation of Presidential Doc-
        uments,* 12.13
    yearbooks, 11.37

units of measure, 2.16–17, 2.64, 3.31
unpublished manuscripts
    abbreviations for types of, 2.19
    citation of, 2.45, 4.19, 10.16, 11.54
    collections, 4.15, 4.20, 8.131–32, 10.16
    facsimiles in appendix, 1.44
unpublished material
    authorship, 8.131
    citation of, 8.83, 8.130–32, 11.52–57
    dissertations as, 8.130, 11.55
    government documents, 12.19
    information services, 8.139
    interviews, 11.49–50
    lectures and speeches, 8.130
    letters, 8.130
    musical scores, 11.58
    reports and proceedings, 11.36
    See also unpublished manuscripts
USSR, 2.13

vector graphics, 13.21–22
videorecordings, 8.145, 11.61
virgule, in poetry, 5.8
viz., 2.26
volume (measure), 2.16–17
volume number, 8.74–83, 8.92, 8.101,
    8.104, 11.14–15. *See also* multivol-
    ume works
vs., 2.26

*Weekly Compilation of Presidential Docu-
    ments,* 12.13
weight, 2.16–17
word division. *See* division of words
word processing programs. *See* computer
    programs
words. *See* division of words; compound
    words; spelling
works of art, 8.147, 11.63–64

year
    comma in, 2.49, 2.66
    in dates, 2.40–51
    era, 2.56
    inclusive numbers, 2.67
    journals, 8.101
yearbooks, 11.37–38

zero, 2.36, 2.40, 6.43–44
zip codes, 2.66, 3.75